RESILIENT HEALTH CARE

Ashgate Studies in Resilience Engineering

Series Editors

Professor Erik Hollnagel, *University of Southern Denmark, Denmark*

Professor Sidney Dekker, *Griffith University, Australia*

Dr Christopher P. Nemeth, *Principal Scientist and Group Leader for Cognitive Systems Engineering, Klein Associates Division, (KAD) of Applied Research Associates (ARA), Dayton, Ohio, USA*

Dr Yushi Fujita, *Technova, Inc., Japan*

Resilience engineering has become a recognized alternative to traditional approaches to safety management. Whereas these have focused on risks and failures as the result of a degradation of normal performance, resilience engineering sees failures and successes as two sides of the same coin – as different outcomes of how people and organizations cope with a complex, underspecified and therefore partly unpredictable environment.

Normal performance requires people and organizations at all times to adjust their activities to meet the current conditions of the workplace, by trading-off efficiency and thoroughness and by making sacrificing decisions. But because information, resources and time are always finite such adjustments will be approximate and consequently performance is variable. Under normal conditions this is of little consequence, but every now and then – and sometimes with a disturbing regularity – the performance variability may combine in unexpected ways and give rise to unwanted outcomes.

The Ashgate Studies in Resilience Engineering series promulgates new methods, principles and experiences that can complement established safety management approaches. It provides invaluable insights and guidance for practitioners and researchers alike in all safety-critical domains. While the Studies pertain to all complex systems they are of particular interest to high-hazard sectors such as aviation, ground transportation, the military, energy production and distribution, and healthcare.

Resilient Health Care

EDITED BY

ERIK HOLLNAGEL
University of Southern Denmark & Centre for Quality, Region of Southern Denmark

JEFFREY BRAITHWAITE
Australian Institute of Health Innovation at University of New South Wales, Australia

ROBERT L. WEARS
University of Florida Health Science Center, USA

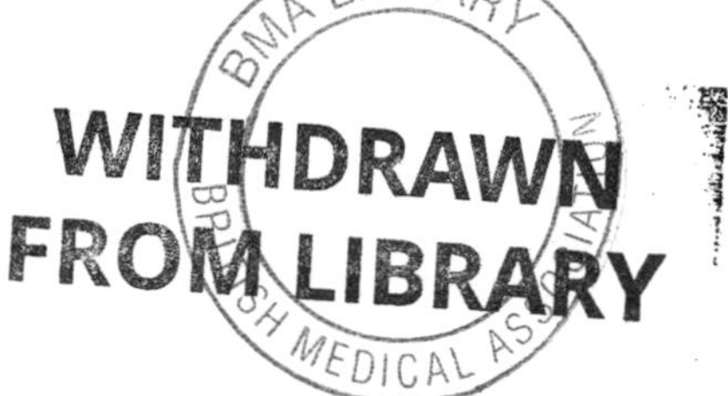

ASHGATE

Published by
Ashgate Publishing Limited
Wey Court East
Union Road
Farnham
Surrey, GU9 7PT
England

Ashgate Publishing Company
110 Cherry Street
Suite 3–1
Burlington, VT 05401-3818
USA

www.ashgate.com

British Library Cataloguing in Publication Data
A catalogue record for this book is available from the British Library.

The Library of Congress has cataloged the printed edition as follows:
Hollnagel, Erik, 1941–
Resilient health care / by Erik Hollnagel, Jeffrey Braithwaite and Robert L. Wears.
pages cm. – (Ashgate studies in resilience engineering)
Includes bibliographical references and index.
ISBN 978-1-4094-6978-0 (hardback : alk. paper) – ISBN 978-1-4094-6979-7 (ebook) – ISBN 978-1-4094-6980-3 (epub)
1. Health services administration. 2. Health facilities – Administration. 3. Sustainable development. 4. Organizational effectivenes. I. Braithwaite, Jeffrey, 1954– II. Wears, Robert L. III. Title.

RA971.H573 2013
362.1068–dc23

2013018027

ISBN 9781409469780 (hbk)
ISBN 9781409469797 (ebk – PDF)
ISBN 9781409469803 (ebk – ePUB)

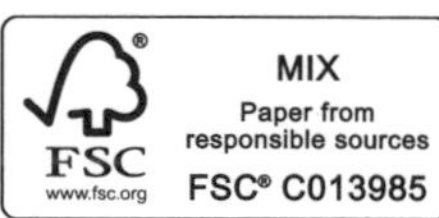

Printed in the United Kingdom by Henry Ling Limited,
at the Dorset Press, Dorchester, DT1 1HD

Contents

List of Figures and Tables

Figures

Tables

List of Contributors

René Amalberti is professor of medicine, MD, PhD. After a residency in psychiatry, he entered the Air Force in 1977, graduating in aerospace medicine, and became professor of medicine in 1995. In the late 1990s, he moved his focus of research to patient safety, retiring in 2007. He is now senior advisor of patient safety at the Haute Autorité de Santé and head of prevention strategies at a private medical insurance company (MACSF). He has published over 100 international papers and chapters, and authored or co-authored ten books on human error, violations, risk management and system safety in various professional environments.

Adélaïde Blavier obtained her PhD in psychology in 2006. With a background in neuropsychology and cognitive psychology, her research concerns visual perception and, more particularly, ocular movements and depth perception in relation to human error within complex systems transformed by the introduction of new technologies. Her previous research was conducted in the medical domain, particularly in minimal access surgery. Dr Blavier's current research focuses on the relations between visual memory and ocular movement in expert activity (driving, medical images, art history and abstract paintings).

William Bond, MD, MS, currently serves as medical director of the Lehigh Valley Health Network (LVHN) Interdisciplinary Simulation Center. He initiated simulation efforts to improve patient safety throughout LVHN, including in situ, procedural, and inter-professional simulation. Mr Bond serves as the designated institutional official for LVHN, a liaison role to the ACGME. He has published on topics related to patient safety, resident education, cognitive error, and differential diagnostic reasoning.

Jeffrey Braithwaite, BA, MIR (Hons), MBA, DipLR, PhD, FAIM, FCHSM, is foundation director of the Australian Institute of Health Innovation, director of the Centre for Clinical Governance Research and a professor in the Faculty of Medicine, University of New South Wales, Australia. His research examines the changing nature of health systems, attracting funding of more than AU$55 million. Dr Braithwaite has published over 500 publications. He has presented at, or chaired, international and national conferences on more than 500 occasions, including over 60 keynote addresses. He has won many awards for his research and teaching. Further details are available on his Wikipedia entry at http://en.wikipedia.org/wiki/Jeffrey_Braithwaite.

Karen Cardiff, BScN, MSc, MHSc, is a health services researcher at the School of Population and Public Health, University of British Columbia. Her particular interest lies in understanding how safety is created and maintained in complex adaptive systems such as health care. Karen holds degrees in nursing (University of British Columbia), community health and epidemiology (University of Toronto), and human factors and system safety (Lund University).

Sheuwen Chuang has more than 20 years' experience with the aerospace industry, IT and health care industries. She is CEO of the Health Policy and Care Research Center and an assistant professor at the School of Health Care Administration of the Taipei Medical University, Taiwan. Her research interests lie in the area of health policy and quality / safety management in different health care system levels. She also teaches systems thinking in health care, both on graduate and undergraduate courses.

Robyn Clay-Williams, BEng, PhD, is a post-doctoral fellow in the field of human factors in health care at the Australian Institute of Health Innovation, University of New South Wales, Australia. She spent 24 years with the Royal Australian Air Force, where she worked as an electronics engineer, flight instructor and test pilot. Her PhD investigated attitude and behavioural changes in multi-disciplinary health care teams resulting from the implementation of a crew resource management (CRM) intervention. Dr Clay-

Williams's specific areas of interest in health care include resilience, teams and teamwork, system dynamics modelling, simulation, and usability test and evaluation of medical devices and IT systems.

Richard Cook is professor of Healthcare System Safety and chairman of the Department of Patient Safety in the Skolan för teknik och hälsa (School of Technology and Health) in Stockholm, Sweden. After working in the computer industry in supercomputer system design and engineering applications, he received his MD from the University of Cincinnati in 1986. Between 1987 and 1991 he researched expert human performance in anesthesiology and industrial and systems engineering at The Ohio State University. From November 1994 to March 2012, he was a practising anesthesiologist, teacher, and researcher in the Department of Anesthesia and Intensive Care, University of Chicago. Professor Cook is an internationally recognized expert on medical accidents, complex system failures, and human performance at the sharp end of these systems. He has investigated a variety of problems in such diverse areas as urban mass transportation, semiconductor manufacturing, and military software systems, and is often a consultant for not-for-profit organizations, government agencies, and academic groups.

Rollin J. (Terry) Fairbanks, MD, MS, leads the National Center for Human Factors in Healthcare and the Simulation and Training Environment Laboratory, both part of the MedStar Institute for Innovation in Washington, DC. He holds academic appointments as associate professor of emergency medicine at Georgetown University and adjunct associate professor of industrial systems engineering, University at Buffalo. He practises as an attending emergency physician at the MedStar Washington Hospital Center in Washington, DC. A trained human factors engineer, Professor Fairbanks focuses on applying the principles of safety science to the health care industry.

Alessandra Gorini, MA, PhD, obtained her candidate diploma in experimental psychology in 2001 with a thesis on the functional neuroimaging of reasoning processes. In 2004, she obtained a

Masters in clinical neuropsychology at the University of Padua. She obtained a second master (2006) and a PhD in affective neuroscience (2010) in Maastricht. Dr Gorini has a research position at the University of Milan, where she studies decision-making processes from a cognitive perspective. She is author of more than 40 scientific papers published on indexed peer-reviewed international journals, and two monographs.

Erik Hollnagel, PhD, is chief consultant at the Center for Quality, Region of Southern Denmark, professor at the University of Southern Denmark (DK) and emeritus professor at the University of Linköping, Sweden. He has worked at universities, research centres, and industries in Denmark, England, Norway, Sweden and France, focusing on problems from many domains, including nuclear power generation, aerospace and aviation, software engineering, land-based traffic, and healthcare. His professional interests include industrial safety, resilience engineering, patient safety, accident investigation, and understanding large-scale socio-technical systems. Dr Hollnagel has published widely and is the author / editor of 20 books – including four books on resilience engineering – as well as a large number of papers and book chapters. His latest titles are: *FRAM – the Functional Resonance Analysis Method, Governance and Control of Financial Systems, Resilience Engineering in Practice: A Guidebook* and *The ETTO Principle: Why Things that Go Right, Sometimes Go Wrong*.

Nicolas Lot has a PhD in sociology of organizations (2008). His research topic was the dynamic of ambiguity in the nuclear power plant. Over eight years, he performed many observations and analyses in various situations. His main expertise concerns the nuclear sector and collective reliability around the relationship of teams with rules, and the consideration of the cultural and identity dimensions. Dr Lot works for Dédale, France.

Carl Macrae is a social psychologist specialising in how organisations achieve high levels of safety and resilience. His current work as a health foundation improvement science fellow examines the role of regulation in patient safety improvement. Dr Macrae is a senior research fellow in the Centre for Patient

Safety and Service Quality, Imperial College, London, and a research associate at the Centre for Analysis of Risk and Regulation, London School of Economics. He worked previously as special advisor at the NHS National Patient Safety Agency, in the regulatory risk group of an investment bank. Dr Macrae completed his doctorate in collaboration with a major airline.

Ketti Mazzocco is research fellow at the Department of Decision Sciences, Bocconi University in Milan, and contract consultant for eCancer Medical Science. She holds a bachelor degree in psychology from the University of Padua, Italy, a PhD in cognitive science from the same institution and a degree in systemic therapy at the Milan Center for Family Therapy. Dr Mazzocco's contributions include studies on bounded rationality in economics, medical decision making and communication for health promotion. Her main research interests are in the field of reasoning and decision under risk and uncertainty, with particular attention to emotions and individual differences as predictive factors of choices and information processing. Recently, particular attention has been given to patient empowerment, combining cognitive findings and methodologies with a systemic approach.

Peter Nugus, MA Hons, MEd, PhD, is assistant professor in the Centre for Medical Education and the Department of Family Medicine at McGill University, Montreal, Canada. He is a sociologist whose ethnographic research – in emergency departments and various acute and community settings – has focused on workplace and organisational learning, care coordination, and culture and identity in complex organizations. Dr Nugus has publications in leading journals and has been awarded competitive grants, and Fulbright and Australian Government Endeavour Scholarships. He has been a post-doctoral scholar at the University of New South Wales (where he undertook his PhD), UCLA, Columbia University and the Netherlands Institute for Health Services Research.

Anne-Sophie Nyssen is professor of cognitive ergonomics and work psychology at the University of Liege, Belgium. Since 2003, she has headed a small research team specialising in two main areas: the study of human error, human reliability, cognitive processes and the assessment of new technology at work. For the last ten years, Professor Nyssen has contributed to the development and use of simulations for training and research in medical expertise. Central to the team's lab is the use of multiple techniques to collect data in order to understand the complexity of work systems: observation of performance and interviews in real work contexts, in simulated situations and lab settings.

Jean Pariès graduated from the French National School of Civil Aviation as an engineer then joined the DGAC dealing with air safety regulations. He has been a member of the ICAO Human Factors and Flight Safety Study Group since its creation in 1988. In 1990, he joined the Bureau Enquêtes Accident as deputy head and head of investigations, leading the technical investigation into the Mont Saint-Odile air accident in 1992. In 1994, he left the BEA to become a founding member (and now CEO) of Dédale SA. Based in Paris and Melbourne, Australia, Dédale's activity focuses on the human and organisational dimensions of safety, for aviation as well as for nuclear, railway, hospital, road, and maritime operations. Jean Pariès is a member of the Resilience Engineering core group, and the author of numerous papers, book chapters and communications on human factors in safety. He holds a commercial pilot's licence with instrument, multi-engines, turboprop, and instructor ratings and a helicopter private pilot's licence.

Shawna Perry, MD, is director for patient safety system engineering at Virginia Commonwealth University Health Systems in Richmond, Virginia (USA), and associate professor / associate chair for the Department of Emergency Medicine. Professor Perry's primary research interest is patient safety, with an emphasis on human factors / ergonomics and system failure. She has published widely on topics related to these areas, as well as transitions in care, the impact of IT upon clinical care and naturalistic decision-making.

Jennifer Plumb, BA (Hons), MSc, is a PhD candidate at the Australian Institute of Health Innovation, University of New South Wales, Sydney, Australia. She has previously worked in mental health policy and knowledge management in the United Kingdom National Health Service, and has an academic background in medical anthropology. Her current research interest is in the ethnographic exploration of patient safety in mental health care, particularly as it emerges in multiple forms as a socio-material achievement during everyday professional practice.

Gabriella Pravettoni obtained a MS in experimental psychology at the University of Padua in 1991, and a PhD in cognitive science at the University of Pavia in 1995. After that, she moved to the University of California, Los Angeles (USA), for her post-doctorate in cognitive science. She is at present full professor of cognitive science at the University of Milan, director of the Interdisciplinary Research Center on Decision Making Processes, and coordinator of the post-degree course on cognitive sciences and decision making, University of Milan. Her main interests include the study of cognitive processes, cognitive ergonomics, decision making, patient empowerment and health psychology. Professor Pravettoni is author of many scientific papers on peer-review international journals and of various books on decision making.

Rob Robson, MDCM, MSc, FRCP(C), is the principal advisor for Healthcare System Safety and Accountability in Canada and recently served as the Winnipeg Regional Health Authority's chief patient safety officer for six years. He is a trained healthcare mediator, having worked for more than 15 years in this field. Doctor Robson is a specialist emergency physician who continues to practise, and assistant professor in the Department of Community Health Sciences, University of Manitoba's Faculty of Medicine. He is interested in trying to direct traffic at the tangled intersection of complexity science, conflict engagement, accountability, and patient safety.

Fanny Rome graduated from the French school Ecole Centrale de Lyon in 1995 as an engineer and has a PhD in psychology and ergonomics (2009). Her research topic was the use of work analysis in the aviation safety, where she studied the use of two analysis methods (CREAM and FRAM). Over five years, she performed many observations and analyses in various situations (new aircraft design, event analysis, preparation for takeoff, pilots–controller simulations). Dr Rome joined Dédale, France, as a human factors consultant in 2009 and has, over the last three years, worked on several projects in aviation and healthcare. Her work is focused on research (safety management systems modelling), the collection of data in the field (observations and interviews) and safety training.

Sam Sheps, MD, MSc, FRCP(C), is professor at the School of Population and Public Health, University of British Columbia. He is a health services researcher and was a member of the British Columbia team collecting data from the Canadian Adverse Events Study. Other funded patient safety project work include a Health Canada project assessing approaches to governance and safety in non-health industries, a Canadian Patient Safety Institute-funded study on high reliability in health care and, more recently, a Canadian Health Services Research Foundation-funded study of new approaches to critical incident investigation, applying the concept of resilience engineering to health care.

Patricia H. Strachan, PhD, is an associate professor in the School of Nursing at McMaster University, Canada. She completed a post-doctoral fellowship for cardiovascular nursing research from the Heart and Stroke Foundation of Ontario, Canada. Her research broadly focuses on communication issues involving patients with advanced heart failure and end-of-life planning and care. She is currently applying complexity science to research related to these concepts. Dr Strachan is an investigator with the Canadian Researchers at the End of Life Network (CARENET), in association with Technology Evaluation in the Elderly Network, one of the government of Canada's Networks of Centres of Excellence.

Kathleen M. Sutcliffe is the Gilbert and Ruth Professor of Business Administration and professor of management and organizations at the Stephen M. Ross School of Business, University of Michigan, USA. Her research investigates how organisations and their members cope with uncertainty and unexpected events, and how complex organisations can be designed to be more reliable and resilient. She has served on the editorial boards of the *Academy of Management Journal, Organization Science, Organization Studies,* and currently the *International Public Management Journal.* Books include *Medical Error: What Do We Know? What Do We Do?* (2002), co-edited with Marilynn Rosenthal, and *Managing the Unexpected,* co-authored with Karl Weick (2001, 2007).

Didier Tassaux is a medical doctor. Since 1997, he has worked in the intensive care unit of the University Hospital of Geneva, Switzerland. His area of research is focused on health safety management, basically studying organisational and human factors in anaesthesiology and intensive care. In association with Jean Pariès (CEO of Dédale SA), he performed a study aimed at characterising the resilience features of the biggest intensive care unit in Switzerland. At the same time, Dr Tassaux is following a professional masters course in health care safety management at the Institute for an Industrial Safety Culture (ICSI), in partnership with the Polytechnic National Institute of Toulouse, France.

Charles A. Vincent, M Phil, PhD, is professor of clinical safety research, Department of Surgery and Cancer, Imperial College London. He trained as a clinical psychologist and worked in the British NHS for several years. He established the Clinical Risk Unit at University College in 1995, where he was professor of psychology, before moving to the Department of Surgery and Cancer at Imperial College in 2002. He is the editor of *Clinical Risk Management* (2nd edn, 2001), author of *Patient Safety* (2nd edn 2010) and author of many papers on risk, safety and medical error. From 1999 to 2003, he was a commissioner on the UK Commission for Health Improvement and he has advised on patient safety in many enquiries and committees. In 2007, Dr Vincent was appointed director of the National Institute of Health Research Centre for Patient Safety and Service Quality, Imperial College Healthcare Trust.

Justin Waring is professor of organisational sociology at Nottingham University Business School, UK. His research makes connections between medical sociology and organisational studies in order to develop new theoretical and conceptual perspectives on organisational safety, risk and learning. He has worked in the area of patient safety for over 10 years, and has been at the forefront of research on the socio-cultural analysis of safety and risk.

Robert L. Wears, MD, MS, PhD, is an emergency physician, professor of emergency medicine at the University of Florida, and visiting professor at the Clinical Safety Research Unit, Imperial College, London. He serves on the board of directors of the Emergency Medicine Patient Safety Foundation, and multiple editorial boards, including *Annals of Emergency Medicine, Human Factors and Ergonomics*, the *Journal of Patient Safety*, and the *International Journal of Risk and Safety in Medicine*. He has co-edited two books: *Patient Safety in Emergency Medicine*, and *Resilient Healthcare*. His research interests include technical work studies, resilience engineering, and patient safety as a social movement.

Karl E. Weick is the Rensis Likert Distinguished University Professor of Organizational Behavior and Psychology, and emeritus professor of psychology at the University of Michigan, USA. He joined the Michigan faculty in 1988, after previous faculty positions at the University of Texas, Cornell University, University of Minnesota, and Purdue University. He is a former editor of the journal *Administrative Science Quarterly* (1977–1985), former associate editor of the journal *Organizational Behavior and Human Performance* (1971–1977), and former topic editor for human factors at the journal *Wildfire*. Books include *The Social Psychology of Organizing* (1969, 1979); *Sense-making in Organizations* (1995); and *Managing the Unexpected*, co-authored with Kathleen Sutcliffe (2001, 2007).

Preface: On the Need for Resilience in Health Care

Erik Hollnagel, Jeffrey Braithwaite and Robert L. Wears

This book provides the first comprehensive description of *resilient health care*, henceforth referred to as RHC. Since there are probably only a few who, at the time of publication, have a clear idea about what this means, some words of introduction are appropriate. The simple explanation is that RHC is the application of the concepts and methods of resilience engineering to the field of health care, and in particular to the problems of patient safety. A more detailed explanation and exemplification are provided in the chapters that follow.

The motivation for RHC is threefold, as explained in this preface. The first is the sorry state of affairs in health care. The second is that attempts to improve this so far have had limited success. The third is the potential offered by resilience engineering as an alternative approach to safety and safety management.

The Sorry State of Affairs

The 'sorry state of affairs' of patient safety care is an expression of the fact that the general situation is not acceptable. Care is simply not as safe as it ought to be. To paraphrase Shakespeare, we may say that 'there is something rotten in the state of health care.' Justification for this view is not hard to find, but a few examples will suffice for the present. In a paper appropriately entitled 'Is health care getting safer?' Vincent et al. (2008) noted that 10 per cent of patients admitted to hospitals in the United Kingdom were subject to iatrogenic harm. This level of harm has been found wherever studies of care, via medial record review or other methods, have been conducted. And depending on how iatrogenia is measured, adverse events may occur in every third or fourth admission (Landrigan et al., 2010). In addition, a RAND study by McGlynn et al. (2003) showed poor adherence to many recommended clinical practices, with only 55 per cent of patients receiving care deemed to be appropriate. Almost 10 years after RAND, and in Australia rather than the United States, Runciman and colleagues (2012a; 2012b) found the proportion of patients receiving appropriate levels of care remained at a similar level, this time 57 per cent. There is clearly room for systemic improvement, to put it mildly.

This 'sorry state of affairs' has been recognised for some time, since several large studies in the USA, UK, and Australia as far back as 1955 provided 'clear evidence that medical error is a common and sometimes preventable fact of the delivery of care in several highly developed and well-funded healthcare systems' (Baker and Norton, 2001). We agree with this statement, except that we would substitute 'often' for 'sometimes'. The clincher was the landmark report 'To Err is Human' from the Institute of Medicine in the USA (Kohn, Corrigan and Donaldson, 2000), which made clear that a majority of adverse events were due to systemic faults rather than to individual incompetence (cf. also Chapter 2).

That these circumstances have arisen and that they persist in sophisticated, well-resourced health systems can be attributed to a number of overarching factors. One is that the demand for care is rising because of population ageing. It is also rising because the provision of care is increasingly intense and complicated due largely to inter-linked factors such as technological, diagnostic and therapeutic advances. Another is that opportunities to provide the right care to the right patient at the right time are diminishing because of work pressures and associated demands on clinicians, exacerbated by workforce shortages and ageing workers. A third is the rising costs that are spiralling in many countries, perhaps uncontrollably so. According to estimates based on data from OECD Health Data and the World Health Organization, 2010 health care expenditure ranged from 6.28 per cent of GDP in Mexico to 17.6 per cent of GDP in the USA, while the OECD average was 9.5 per cent – with an estimated growth rate of around 4 per cent annually. This is a vast commitment of the world's resources, especially in times of strained budgets and austerity – whether endogenous or exogenous.

The health system thus has to meet several irreconcilable goals – customer demands, performance pressures, work and workforce stresses, and cost challenges – and to meet them simultaneously. Not surprisingly, this creates stressed circumstances and working conditions (for the system and for the people in it) that not only are far from optimal but are in many respects detrimental to providers and patients alike. It is under these conditions of pressure, uncertainty, and risk that people are expected to deliver care which is safe for patients, cost effective, and of high quality. The diminishing capacity to do so is an urgent problem that has triggered many studies and led to many attempts to solve it. Yet progress has been painfully slow – perhaps because we have tried to solve the problem based on the symptoms but without a proper diagnosis.

Crushed Expectations: The Bane of Conventional Solutions

Dissatisfaction with system performance levels is not unique to health care, but is common across industries – and indeed in practically all types of organised human activity. Other industries have throughout their development either experienced calamitous events, such as spectacular accidents and major disasters, or extended periods of intolerable problems, but have in most cases eventually managed to find workable solutions. When dissatisfaction with the performance of the health care system became common in the 1990s, the obvious reaction was therefore to look to other industries that appeared to do better, in the hope that simply imitating what they did would be a panacea – or at least keep the wolves from the door a little longer.

A pivotal point we want to make is that people who championed learning from other industries (aviation, chip manufacturing, etc.) lacked an adequate appreciation either of what these other industries were doing, or why things worked there, or both. Although few will openly admit that they believe in silver bullets, there was in the beginning the hope among many that it would be possible to find quick remedies that could be 'rolled out', which would make all the problems dissolve. (This is affectionately known as 'picking the low-hanging fruit'.)

Dating from the 1970s, health care has, with varying degrees of optimism and conviction, tried putative solutions such as intensifying bureaucracy, quality circles, quality assurance, root cause analysis, 'lean manufacturing', standardised therapeutic programmes via clinical guidelines, teamwork, use of check-lists, accreditation, and above all, information technology (IT) in various forms. Most times solutions have been introduced in local settings or systems by convinced champions with much enthusiasm but with little or no thought about the principles and values underlying their efforts, or how the initiatives would fit together strategically or, indeed, how they would affect the existing equilibrium. An under-recognised common feature of such initiatives is that they practically represent a highly rationalised, Taylorist approach that presumes predictability and an inherent linearity and proportionality of causes and effects. This is regrettably nowhere to be found in the real world of care delivery. Health systems are not simplistic production lines for car assembly or mining operations for mineral extraction, and can therefore not be precisely described, specified, codified, mechanised, and controlled. Even staunch health care supporters have gradually realised that real progress will require abandoning the Taylorist approach. Indeed, Berwick (2003) has indicated that: '... prevailing strategies rely largely on outmoded theories of control and standardization of work.' It seems to be a cornerstone of the human condition that people believe – or want to believe – that they will be able to solve today's problems, improve things, reduce errors, and ameliorate harm – all with just a few more resources, a bit more effort, another set of recommendations from a wise enquiry, a little more knowledge of the amount and rate of harm being delivered, increasingly precise measurements of system features, tightening up practices or a new whizz-bang IT system that is just around the corner.

It would, of course, be encouraging, even gratifying, if one could see that the accumulated experience had gradually led to a changing perspective – or even better, demonstrable systems improvements. However, there seems to be little system-wide improvement experience, perhaps because most solutions have been applied opportunistically and piecemeal, based on a trial-and-error 'philosophy' (Hollnagel, 1993). With opportunistic control, solutions are chosen because they look good but without much purposeful exploration. If they succeed, they have limited effect, leading to intermittent and localised gains. They can cause more harm than good, suffer unanticipated consequences and burn a lot of money in the process. When they fail, they are simply abandoned; and because they were not chosen for a clear reason, there would be little to learn from the failure. Indeed, project-itis and faddism are rife in health care.

Solutions based on the use of IT have, since the turn of the century, tended to be looked at with unbridled – although generally unfounded – optimism. We can thus find statements like: 'It is widely believed that, when designed and used appropriately, health IT can help create an ecosystem of safer care ...' (Institute of Medicine, 2012). The recently published document 'Health Information Technology Patient Safety Action & Surveillance Plan for Public Comment', published by the Department of Health and Human Services in the USA, defines two health IT patient safety objectives, namely *Use health IT to make care safer*, and *Continuously improve the safety of health IT*. While few would disagree with these, the unspoken assumption is that health IT is a (or the?) solution to the problems, even though health IT is mostly a label. A closer look at actual experiences from other industries might be advised.

One of the lessons that could have been learned, had anyone bothered to make an effort, is that most presumed solutions – with IT being no exception – tend to make the health system more complex and less tractable. Regardless of whether a solution is added to the system as something new or substitutes for something that is already present, it will affect what already goes on in ways that can be difficult to anticipate or even imagine. The assumption that solutions are neutral in their effects and that their introduction into a system therefore only has intended and no unintended consequences is palpably false. Several of the chapters in this book address this issue. The growing complexity shows itself in additional sub-systems, in compliance costs, in quality and safety programs, in bureaucracy, in clinical technology, in IT, and the like. At the very least, we must make a concerted effort to tease out the nature of this growing complexity, and take steps to understand health care as a complex adaptive system (cf. Chapter 6).

Resilience Engineering

In the rush to find 'implementation-amenable', readily-packaged solutions to the undeniable raft of problems in health care, the focus turned to what other industries had done under similar conditions in the past. Little attention was paid to the fact that a number of these other industries, such as nuclear, aviation, and offshore activities, had gradually started to revise their own approach to safety, prompted by the realisation that the tried and trusted methods of the past, which were always limited anyway, were no longer adequate for the present, and would be even less so in the future. One important insight was that *adverse events increasingly needed to be explained as unfortunate combinations of a number of conditions*, rather than as failures of single functions or components – including 'human error'. Another was that *failures should be seen as the flip side of successes*, in the sense that there was no need to evoke special failure mechanisms to explain the former. Both failures and successes have their origin in performance variability on individual and systemic levels. It is just as wrong to attribute successes to careful planning and diligence as it is to attribute failures to incompetence or error. Instead, both owe their occurrence to a mostly unpredictable, but not unimaginable, combination of a number of system characteristics.

The term 'resilience engineering' was put forward to represent this new way of thinking about safety (Hollnagel, Woods and Leveson, 2006), and quickly became recognised as a valuable complement to the established approaches to industrial safety – and soon also to patient safety. Enlightened thinkers in both industry and academia began to appreciate that resilience engineering provided an articulated basis for confronting the puzzles of such phenomena as complexity, interconnectedness, 'system of systems', and ultra-high reliability. The concepts and principles of resilience engineering have since the beginning been continuously refined by applications in such fields as air traffic management, nuclear power generation, offshore production, commercial fishing, and accident investigation. Over time there has been a dawning realisation that resilience is neither limited to handling threats and disturbances, nor confined to situations where something can go wrong. Today, resilience is understood more broadly as the intrinsic ability of a system to adjust its functioning prior to, during, or following changes and disturbances, so that it can sustain required operations under both expected and unexpected conditions. This definition emphasises the ability to continue functioning, rather than simply to react and recover from disturbances, as well as the ability to exploit opportunities that arise, rather than simply survive threats.

Toward Resilient Health Care

In line with this way of thinking, resilient health care can be defined as the ability of the health care system to adjust its functioning prior to, during, or following changes and disturbances, so that it can sustain required performance under both expected and unexpected conditions. In order to strive for health care resilience, it is therefore necessary to study and understand how health systems work, and not just to perpetuate the predominating myopic focus on how they fail. This realisation has led to the juxtaposition of two views on safety, Safety-I and Safety-II, which permeates this book. (The two views are presented in detail in Chapter 1.) Briefly stated, Safety-I is defined by the (relative) absence of adverse events (accidents, incidents). Safety-I is reactive, and assumes that safety can be achieved by first finding, and then eliminating, or weakening, the causes of adverse events. As a contrast to this way of thinking, Safety-II is defined as the ability to succeed under varying conditions, so that the number of intended and acceptable outcomes (in other words, everyday activities) is as high as possible. Where Safety-I focuses on what goes wrong, Safety-II focuses on what goes right, and the purpose of safety management is to achieve and maintain that ability. The importance of making this distinction and its practical consequences are amply illustrated by the chapters that follow.

In agreement with this distinction, and in order to examine various facets of RHC, the book is structured in three parts. Part I, entitled 'Health Care as a Multiple Stakeholder, Multiple Systems

Enterprise', articulates the scope and depth of RHC and the players involved with it. This section highlights the complexities, adaptive capacity and self-organisational features of health care. It provides a context for knowledge and perspectives about the nature of the health system and how it can be conceptualised, particularly emphasising its complexity, patient safety and the quality of care, in the light of the Safety-I, Safety-II dichotomy. Part II, 'The Locus of Resilience – Individuals, Groups, Systems', sharpens the focus, providing a microscope to display the detailed conditions under which resilience manifests itself at differing levels and in characteristic ways. Building on the earlier chapters, Part III, 'The Nature and Practice of Resilient Health Care', then scrutinises ways of 'being' resilient, and 'doing' resilience, in everyday activities. Finally, in the Epilogue, the book synthesises key learning points and implications for various stakeholder groups interested in health care resilience.

PART I
Health Care as a Multiple Stakeholder, Multiple Systems Enterprise

Chapter 1
Making Health Care Resilient: From Safety-I to Safety-II

Erik Hollnagel

Safety as the Freedom From Unacceptable Risk

Safety has traditionally been defined as a condition where nothing goes wrong. Or rather, since we know that it is impossible to ensure that nothing goes wrong, as a condition where the number of things that go wrong is acceptably small – whatever 'acceptably' may mean. This is, however, an indirect and somewhat paradoxical definition since safety is defined by what it is not, by what happens when it is missing, rather than by what it is. One consequence of this definition is that safety is measured indirectly, not by its presence or as a quality in itself, but by the consequences of its absence.

In relation to human activity it makes good practical sense to focus on situations where things go wrong, both because such situations by definition are unexpected and because they may lead to unintended and unwanted harm or loss of life and property. Throughout the ages, the starting point for safety concerns has therefore been the occurrence, potential or actual, of some kind of adverse outcome, whether it has been categorised as a risk, a hazard, a near miss, an incident, or an accident. Historically speaking, new types of accidents have been accounted for by the introduction of new types of causes (e.g. metal fatigue, 'human error,' organisational failure) rather than by challenging or changing the basic underlying assumption of causality. We have, therefore, through centuries become so accustomed to explaining accidents in terms of cause–effect relations – simple or compound – that we no longer notice it. And we cling tenaciously to this tradition, although it has becomes increasingly difficult to reconcile with reality.

Habituation

An unintended but unavoidable consequence of associating safety with things that go wrong is a creeping lack of attention to things that go right. The psychological explanation for that is called habituation, a form of adaptive behaviour that can be described as non-associative learning. Through habituation we learn to disregard things that happen regularly, simply because they happen regularly. In academic psychology, habituation has been studied at the level of neuropsychology and also has usually been explained at that level (Thompson and Spencer, 1966).

It is, however, entirely possible also to speak about habituation at the level of everyday human behaviour (actions and responses). This was noted as far back as 1890, when William James, one of the founding fathers of psychology, wrote that 'habit diminishes the conscious attention with which our acts are performed' (James, 1890: 114). In today's language it means that we stop paying attention to something as soon as we get used to doing it. After some time, we neither notice that which goes smoothly nor do we think it is necessary to do so. This applies both to actions and their outcomes – both what we do ourselves and what others do.

From an evolutionary perspective, as well as from the point of view of an efficiency-thoroughness trade-off (Hollnagel, 2009a), habituation makes a lot of sense. While there are good reasons to pay attention to the unexpected and the unusual, it may be a waste of time and effort to pay much attention to that which is common or similar. To quote James again: 'Habitual actions are certain, and being in no danger of going astray from their end, need no extraneous help' (p. 149). Reduced attention is precisely what happens when actions regularly produce the intended and expected results and when things 'simply' work. When things go right there is no recognisable difference between the expected and the actual, hence nothing that attracts attention or initiates an arousal reaction. Neither is there any motivation to try to understand why things went well: they obviously went well because the system – people and technology – worked as it should and because nothing untoward happened. While the first argument – the lack of a noticeable difference between outcomes – is acceptable, the second argument is fatally flawed. The reason for that will become clear in the following.

Looking at What Goes Wrong Rather Than Looking at What Goes Right

To illustrate the consequences of looking at what goes wrong rather than looking at what goes right, consider Figure 1.1. This represents the case where the (statistical) probability of a failure is 1 out of 10,000 – technically written as $p = 10^{-4}$. This means that for every time we expect that something will go wrong (the thin line), there are 9,999 times where we should expect that things will go right and lead to the outcome we want (the grey area). The ratio of 1:10,000 corresponds to a system or organisation where the emphasis is on performance (cf. Amalberti, 2006); the ratio would be even more extreme for an ultra-safe system. In health care the ratio has for many years been around 1:10, e.g., Carthey, de Leval and Reason (2001).

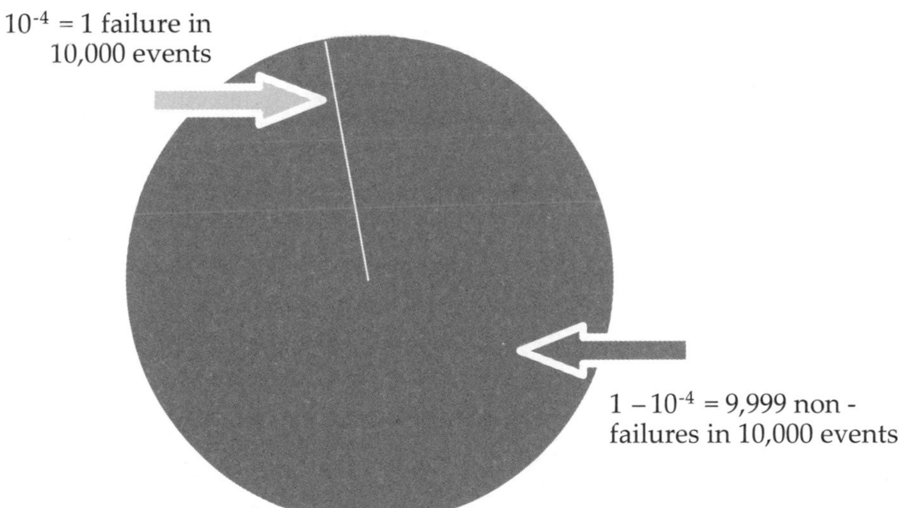
10^{-4} = 1 failure in
10,000 events
$1 - 10^{-4}$ = 9,999 non -
failures in 10,000 events

Figure 1.1 The imbalance between things that go right and things that go wrong

The tendency to focus on what goes wrong is reinforced in many ways. It is often required by regulators and authorities; it is supported by models and methods; it is documented in countless databases and illustrated by almost as many graphs; it is described in literally thousands of papers, books, and conference proceedings; and there are an untold number of experts, consultants, and companies that constantly remind us of the need to avoid risks, failures, and accidents – and of how their services can help to do just that. The net result is abundant information both about how things go wrong and about what must be done to prevent this from happening. The focus on failures also conforms to our stereotypical understanding of what safety is and on how safety should be managed, cf. above. The recipe is the simple principle known as 'find and fix': look for failures and malfunctions, try to find their causes, and try to eliminate causes and / or improve barriers.

One unfortunate and counterproductive consequence of this is that safety and the core activity (treating patients) compete for resources; this means that investments in safety are seen as costs, and therefore (sometimes) hard to justify or sustain. Another consequence is that learning is limited to that which has gone wrong, which means that it only happens infrequently and only uses a fraction of the data available. (A more cynical view is that learning is limited to what we are able to describe and explain.)

The situation is quite different when it comes to that which goes right, i.e., the 9,999 events out of the 10,000. A focus on what goes right receives little encouragement. There is no demand from authorities and regulators to look at what works well, and if someone should want to do so, there is little help to be found; we have few theories or models about how human and organisational performance succeeds, and few methods to help us study how it happens; examples are few and far between (Reason, 2008), and actual data are difficult to locate; it is hard to find papers, books or other forms of scientific literature about it; and there are few people who claim expertise in this area or even consider it worthwhile. Furthermore, it clashes with the traditional focus on failures, and even those who find it a reasonable endeavour are at a loss when it comes to the practicalities: there are no simple methods or tools and very few good examples to learn from.

Yet one interesting consequence of this perspective is that safety and core activity no longer compete for resources; what benefits one will also benefit the other. Another consequence is that learning can focus on that which has gone right, which means that there are literally countless opportunities for learning, and that data are readily available – once the attention is turned away from failures.

Safety-I: Avoiding Things that Go Wrong

The traditional definition of safety as a condition where the number of adverse outcomes (accidents / incidents / near misses) is as low as possible can be called Safety-I. The purpose of managing Safety-I is consequently to achieve and maintain that state. The US Agency for Healthcare Research and Quality, for instance, defines safety as the 'freedom from accidental injury', while the International Civil Aviation Organization defines safety as 'the state in which harm to persons or of property damage is reduced to, and maintained at or below, an acceptable level through a continuing process of hazard identification and risk management.'

The 'philosophy' of Safety-I is illustrated by Figure 1.2. Safety-I promotes a bimodal or binary view of work and activities, according to which they either succeed or fail. When everything works as it should ('normal' functioning), the outcomes will be acceptable; things go right, in the sense that the number of adverse events is acceptably small. But when something goes wrong, when there is a malfunction, human or otherwise, this will lead to a failure (an unacceptable outcome). The issue is therefore how the transition from normal to abnormal (or malfunction) takes, place, e.g., whether it happens through an abrupt or sudden transition or through a gradual 'drift into failure'. According to the logic of Safety-I, safety and efficiency can be achieved if this transition can be blocked. This unavoidably leads to an emphasis on *compliance* in the way work is carried out.

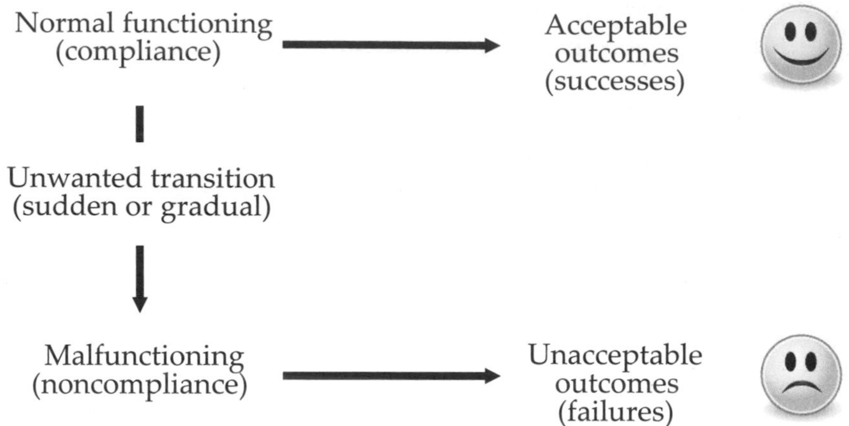

Figure 1.2 The Safety-I view of failures and successes

The focus on failures creates a need to find the causes of what went wrong. When a cause has been found, the next logical step is either to eliminate it or to disable suspected cause–effect links. Following that, the outcome should then be measured by counting how many fewer things go wrong after the intervention. Safety-I thus implies what might be called a 'hypothesis of different causes,' which posits that the causes or 'mechanisms' of adverse events are different from those of events that succeed. If that was not the case, the elimination of such causes and the neutralisation of such 'mechanisms' would also reduce the likelihood that things could go right and hence be counterproductive.

The background for the Safety-I perspective is found in well-understood, well-tested, and well-behaved systems. It is characteristic of such systems that there is a high degree of reliability of equipment, that workers and managers are vigilant in their testing, observations, procedures, training, and operations, that staff are well trained, that management is enlightened, and that good operating procedures are in place. If these assumptions are correct, humans – as 'fallible machines' – are clearly a liability and their performance variability can be seen as a threat. According to the logic of Safety-I, the goal – the coveted state of safety – can be achieved by constraining all kinds of performance variability. Examples of frequently used constraints are selection, strict training, barriers of various kinds, procedures, standardisation, rules, and regulations. The undue optimism in the efficacy of this solution has extended historical roots. But whereas the optimism may have been justified to some extent 100 years ago, it is not so today. The main reason is that the work environment has changed dramatically, and to such an extent that the assumptions of yesteryear are no longer valid.

Safety-I: Reactive Safety Management

The nature of safety management clearly depends on the definition of safety. From a Safety-I perspective, the purpose of safety management is to make sure that the number of adverse outcomes is kept as low as possible – or as low as reasonably practicable (e.g. Melchers, 2001). A good example of that is provided by the WHO research cycle shown in Figure 1.3. The figure shows a repeated cycle of steps that begins when something has gone wrong so that someone has been harmed. In health care, 'measuring harm' means counting how many patients are harmed or killed and from what type of adverse events. In railways, accidents can be defined as 'employee deaths, disabling injuries and minor injuries, per 200,000 hours worked by the employees of the railway company' or 'train and grade crossing accidents that meet the reporting criteria, per million train miles'. Similar definitions can be found in every domain where safety is a concern.

This approach to safety management is *reactive*, because it is based on responding to something that either has gone wrong or has been identified as a risk – as something that could go wrong. The response typically involves looking for ways to eliminate the cause – or causes – that have been found, or to control the risks, either by finding the causes and eliminating them, or by improving options for detection and recovery. Reactive safety management embraces a *causality credo*, which goes as follows: (1) Adverse outcomes (accidents, incidents) happen when something goes wrong. (2) Adverse outcomes therefore have causes, which can be found and treated.

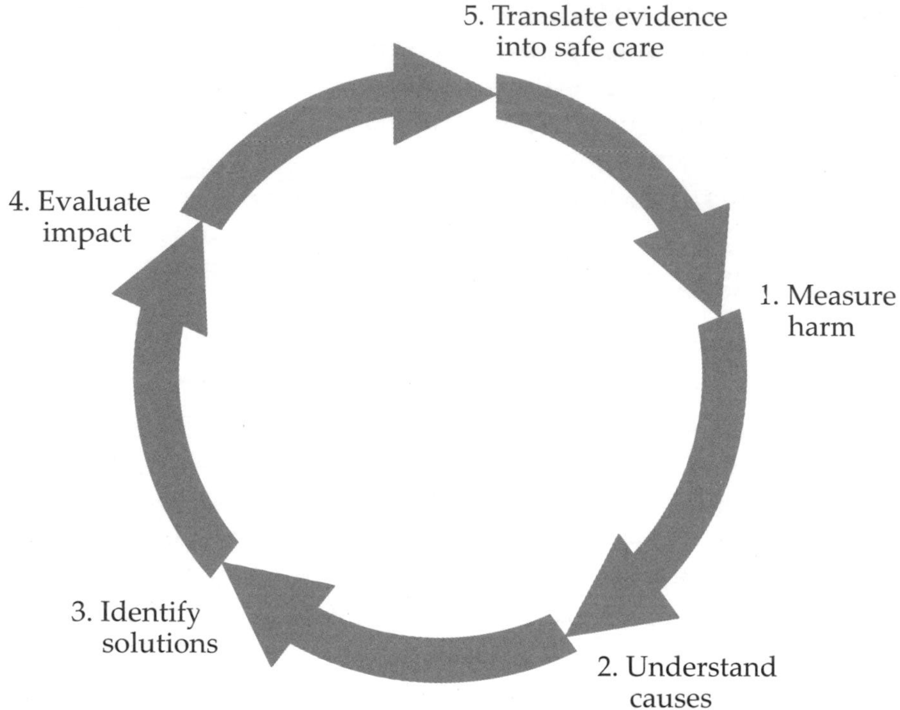

Figure 1.3 Reactive Safety Management Cycle (WHO)

From a Safety-I perspective, the purpose of safety management is to keep the number of accidents and incidents as low as possible by reacting when an unacceptable event has occurred. Such reactive safety management can work in principle if events do not occur so often that it becomes difficult or impossible to take care of the actual work, i.e., the primary activities. But if the frequency of adverse events increases, the need to respond will sooner or later require so much capacity that the reactions both become inadequate and partly lag behind the process. In practice, it means that control of the situation is lost and with that, the ability to manage safety effectively (Hollnagel and Woods, 2005).

Practical examples of this condition are easy to find. If patients are admitted to the emergency room at a rate that is higher than the rate by which they can be treated and discharged, the capacity to treat them will soon be exhausted. This can happen during everyday conditions (Wears, Perry et al., 2006), or during an epidemic (Antonio et al., 2004). On a more mundane level, most health care organisations, as well as most industries, are struggling to keep ahead of a maelstrom of incident reports mandated by law. Even if only the most serious incidents are analysed, there may still be insufficient time to understand and respond to what happened.

Another condition is that the process being managed is familiar and sufficiently regular to allow responses to be prepared ahead of time (anticipation). The worst situation is clearly when something completely unknown happens, since time and resources then must be spent on finding out what it is and work out what to do, before a response can actually be given. In order for reactive safety management to be effective, it must be possible to recognise events so quickly that the organisation can initiate a prepared response with minimal delay. The downside of this is that hasty and careless recognition may lead to inappropriate and ineffective responses.

Safety-II: Ensuring that Things Go Right

As technical and socio-technical systems have continued to develop, not least due to the allure of ever more powerful information technology, systems and work environments have gradually become more intractable (Hollnagel, 2010). Since the models and methods of Safety-I assume that systems are tractable, in the sense that they are well understood and well behaved, Safety-I models and methods are less and less able to deliver the required and coveted 'state of safety.' Because this inability cannot be overcome by 'stretching' the tools of Safety-I even further, it makes sense to consider whether the problem may lie in the definition of safety. One option is, therefore, to change the definition and to focus on what goes right rather than on what goes wrong (as suggested by Figure 1.1). Doing so will change the definition of safety from 'avoiding that something goes wrong' to 'ensuring that everything goes right' – or more precisely, to the ability to succeed under varying conditions, so that the number of intended and acceptable outcomes (in other words, everyday activities) is as high as possible. The consequence of this definition is that the basis for safety and safety management now becomes an understanding of why things go right, which means an understanding of everyday activities.

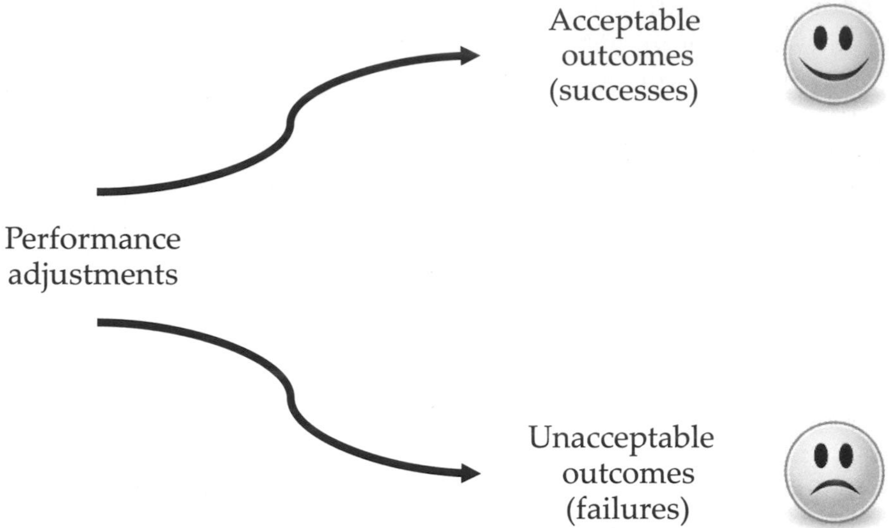

Figure 1.4 The Safety-II view of failures and successes

Safety-II explicitly assumes that systems work because people are able to adjust what they do to match the conditions of work. People learn to identify and overcome design flaws and functional glitches, because they can recognise the actual demands and adjust their performance accordingly, and because they interpret and apply procedures to match the conditions. People can also detect and correct when something goes wrong or when it is about to go wrong, hence they can intervene before the situation becomes seriously worsened. The result of that is performance variability, not in the negative sense where variability is seen as a deviation from some norm or standard, but in the positive sense that variability represents the adjustments that are the basis for safety and productivity (Figure 1.4).

In contrast to Safety-I, Safety-II acknowledges that systems are incompletely understood, that descriptions can be complicated, and that changes are frequent and irregular rather than infrequent and regular. Safety-II, in other words, acknowledges that systems are intractable rather than tractable (Hollnagel, 2010). While the reliability of technology and equipment in such systems may be high, workers and managers frequently trade off thoroughness for efficiency, the competence of staff varies and may be inconsistent or incompatible, and reliable operating procedures are scarce.

Under these conditions, humans are clearly an asset rather than a liability and their ability to adjust what they do to the conditions is a strength rather than a threat.

Performance variability or performance adjustments are a *sine qua non* for the functioning of socio-technical systems, unless they are extremely simple. Unacceptable outcomes or failures can, therefore, not be prevented by eliminating or constraining performance variability, since that would also affect the desired acceptable outcomes. Instead, efforts are needed to support the necessary improvisations and performance adjustments by clearly representing the resources and constraints of a situation and by making it easier to anticipate the consequences of actions. Performance variability should be managed by dampening it if it is going in the wrong direction and amplifying it if is going in the right direction. In order to do so, it is necessary first to acknowledge the presence – and inevitability – of performance variability, second to monitor it, and third to control it. That is the remit of safety management according to Safety-II.

Safety-II: Proactive Safety Management

Safety-II management and resilience engineering both assume that everything basically happens in the same way, regardless of the outcome. This means that there is no need to have one set of causes and 'mechanisms' for things that go wrong (accident and incidents), and another for things that go right (everyday work). The purpose of safety management is to ensure the latter, but by doing so it will also reduce the former. Although Safety-I and Safety-II both lead to a reduction in unwanted outcomes, they use fundamentally different approaches with important consequences for how the process is managed and measured – as well as for productivity and quality.

From a Safety-II perspective, the purpose of safety management is to ensure that as much as possible goes right, in the sense that everyday work achieves its stated purposes. This cannot be done by response alone, since that will only correct what has happened. Safety management must instead be proactive so that adjustments are made *before* something happens and therefore affect how it happens or even prevent something from happening. The main advantage is that early responses, on the whole, require less effort because the consequences of the event will have had less time to develop and spread. And early responses can obviously save valuable time.

For proactive safety management to work, it is necessary to foresee what could happen with acceptable certainty and to have the appropriate means (people and resources) to do something about it. That in turn requires an understanding of how the system works, of how its environment develops and changes, and of how functions may depend on and affect each other. This understanding can be developed by looking for patterns and relations across events rather than for causes of individual events. To see and find those patterns, it is necessary to take time to understand what happens rather than spend all resources on firefighting.

A trivial example is to 'batten down the hatches' when bad weather is approaching. While this expression has its origin in the navy, many people living on land – or on an oilrig – have also learned the value of preparing for a storm. In a different domain, the precautions following the World Health Organization's warning in 2009 of a possible H1N1 flu pandemic are an example of proactive safety management. After the warning was issued, European and other governments began to stockpile considerable amounts of drugs and vaccines to ensure that the necessary resources were in place. Although it later turned out to have been a false alarm, it illustrates the essential features of proactive safety management.

It is obviously a problem for proactive safety management that the future is uncertain and that an expected situation may fail to happen. In that case, preparations will have been made in vain, and time and resources may have been wasted. It is also a problem that predictions may be imprecise or incorrect, so that the wrong preparations are made. Proactive safety management thus requires taking a risk, not least an economic one. But the alternative of not being ready when something serious happens will indubitably be even more expensive in both the short and the long runs.

Conclusion

While day-to-day activities at the sharp end never are reactive only, the pressure in most work situations is to be efficient rather than thorough, and this reduces the possibilities of being proactive (Hollnagel, 2011a). Proactive safety management does require that some effort is spent up-front thinking about what could possibly happen, to prepare appropriate responses, to allocate resources, and make contingency plans. Here are some practical suggestions for how to begin that process:

- *Look at what goes right as well as what goes wrong.* Learn from what succeeds as well as from what fails. Indeed, do not wait for something bad to happen but try to understand what actually takes place in situations where nothing out of the ordinary seems to happen. Things do not go well because people simply follow the procedures. Things go well because people make sensible adjustments according to the demands of the situation. Find out what these adjustments are and try to learn from them!
- *When something has gone wrong, look for everyday performance variability rather than for specific causes.* Whenever something is done, it is a safe bet that it has been tried before. People are quick to find out which performance adjustments work and soon come to rely on them – precisely because they work. Blaming people for doing what they usually do is therefore counterproductive. Instead, one should try to find the performance adjustments people usually make as well as the reasons for them. Things go wrong for the same reasons that they go right, but it is far easier and less incriminating to study how things go right.
- *Look at what happens regularly and focus on events based on how often they happen (frequency) rather than how serious they are (severity).* It is much easier to be proactive for that which happens frequently than for that which happens rarely. A small improvement in everyday performance may be more important than a large improvement in exceptional performance.

- *Allow time to reflect, to learn, and to communicate.* If all the time is used trying to make ends meet, there will no time to consolidate experiences or replenish resources – including how the situation is understood. It must be legitimate within the organisational culture to allocate resources – especially time – to reflect, to share experiences, and to learn. If that is not the case, then how can anything ever improve?
- *Remain sensitive to the possibility of failure – and be mindful.* Try to think of – or even make a list of – undesirable situations and imagine how they may occur. Then think of ways in which they can either be prevented from happening, or be recognised and responded to as they are happening. This is the essence of proactive safety management.

The Way Ahead

What people do in everyday work situations is usually a mixture of Safety-I and Safety-II. The precise balance depends on many things, such as the nature of the work, the experience of the people, the organisational climate, management and customer pressures, etc. Everybody knows that prevention is better than cure, but the conditions may not always be conducive to that.

It is a different matter when it comes to the levels of management and regulatory activities. Here it is clear that the Safety-I view dominates, for reasons that have been explained at the beginning of this chapter. (The imbalance may be due to an efficiency–thoroughness trade-off as well: it is much simpler to count the few events that fail than the many that do not. And it is also – wrongly – assumed to be easier to explain the former rather than the latter.)

Since the socio-technical systems on which our existence depends continue to become more and more complicated, it seems clear that staying with a Safety-I approach will be inadequate in the long; that may by now even be the case also in the short run. Taking a Safety-II approach should therefore not be a difficult choice to make. Yet the way ahead does not lie in a wholesale replacement of Safety-I by Safety-II, but rather in a combination of the two ways of thinking. It is still the case that the majority of adverse events are relatively simple – or can be treated as relatively simple without serious consequences – and that they therefore can be dealt with in the way we have become accustomed to. But there are a growing number of cases where this approach will not work. For these, it is necessary to adopt a Safety-II perspective – which essentially means adopting a resilience engineering perspective. Safety-II is first and foremost a different way of looking at safety, hence also a different way of applying many of the familiar methods and techniques. In addition to that, it will also require methods on its own, to look at things that go right, to analyse how things work, and to *manage* performance variability rather than just *constraining* it.

Chapter 2
Resilience, the Second Story, and Progress on Patient Safety

Richard Cook

The History of *A Tale of Two Stories*

In 1997, there was a small meeting of researchers to explore the scientific basis for making progress on patient safety. The result of that meeting was a monograph (Cook, Woods and Miller, 1998) that proposed that productive insights into safety were likely to come from exploring the 'second story' that lay behind the 'first story' incidents and accidents.

First stories are accounts of 'celebrated' accidents. There are many of these stories and their celebration in the press leads to each being known by a single name or short phrase: the Betsy Lehman case, the Florida wrong leg case, the Ben Kolb case, etc. (Belkin, 1997). The first story inevitably characterises the accident as both a catastrophe and a blunder. The juxtaposition of these two facets makes the first story easy to comprehend and asserts a single causal chain: human error leading directly to injury.

Accounts of accidents are inevitably simplifications of the work world – first stories are constructed to make the accident comprehensible to outsiders. First stories are easy to remember, easy to recount, and – at least apparently – easy to interpret. Because the causal mechanism (human error) is always the same, a collection of first stories leads inevitably to the conclusion that the phenomenon is widespread. Such collections become instruments for asserting that a domain of practice has 'a human error problem'. Eventually the collections reach a critical mass sufficient to evoke political action, which usually takes the form of a resolve to eradicate 'error'.

By the mid-1990s, the human error problem in US health care was garnering significant political attention. The first stories were complemented by a series of studies showing that patients often had bad outcomes solely as a result of their care (cf. Brennan et al., 1991). Some of us anticipated the likely trajectory of political action and wanted to head it off. Experience in domains such as nuclear power generation had shown that efforts to eradicate 'error' would be unproductive. We perceived a risk and opportunity.

The risk was that the nascent patient safety movement would become just another attack on 'human error'. This would delay any real progress on safety for a decade or more. Although sterile, programmatic approaches to eradicating human error are seductive and, at first glance, feasible. The political response, when it came, was likely to be programmatic and could easily misfire. It seemed likely that the energy derived from an 'error crisis in medicine' would be invested in programmes that were easy to understand and implement and that offered immediate returns. Many influential people expressed optimism that 'low-hanging fruit' could easily be harvested to achieve quick improvements to safety. But experience in other domains suggested that making progress would be more expensive, take longer, and ultimately be less successful than the proponents promised.

The opportunity was that, unlike nuclear power and other domains that had become bogged down with error, health care could skip a decade or more of painful learning from disillusion with successive programmatic failures. The health care community could immediately begin with productive work on safety itself.

The agenda for seizing this opportunity was research based. The community of people who had worked on safety in complex technical systems could be mobilised. Work could begin quickly to uncover the core tasks and conflicted conditions that shaped human performance. The competing demands and bulky technology that generated new failure pathways could be identified and characterised. The hedges and gambles that served as strategies for managing the irreducible uncertainty of domains of practice could be inferred. The difficult problems, the messy details, the contingencies that lay underneath the action sequences, could all be made explicit. The deep domain knowledge that drove technical work could be captured, described, and used. The results of these efforts would serve as the basis for the rational, gradual, and deliberate interventions.

The naiveté and hubris of this academic view of the risks and opportunities of the early days of patient safety is, to put it politely, staggering. This academic view took no account of the important economic, social, organisational, professional, and political forces that surround health care. Even well prepared, deliberate changes to such a large, intricate, and contested system are likely to fail; such changes cut across too many agendas and run foul of too many entrenched interests to be successful. Because safety emerges from the interactions between all the elements of the system, efforts to improve it will engage many established agendas and interests. This makes success of patient safety initiatives even less likely than for other sorts of change.

The plan was also mistimed. During the 1990s, public and private actors raised consciousness around patient safety and sought political attention. These activities gradually assembled the public and political interest, reaching the political critical mass needed to force government action at the end of the decade. The late 1999 release of the Institute of Medicine (IOM) report *To Err is Human* (Kohn, Corrigan and Donaldson, 2000), and the Clinton administration's establishment in early 2000 of a task force to coordinate government responses to that report was the result.

Achieving the political critical mass to launch a major government initiative is a significant accomplishment but also one with unavoidable consequences. The chain reaction that follows spends its political energy quickly. In social and political terms this means that only programmatic approaches *already available when the chain reaction begins* can soak up the energy being released. If there had ever been an opportunity to prepare the ground for skipping unproductive efforts to eradicate error, this occurred in the 1980s, not at the end of the 1990s. What appeared to be a risk was actually a forgone conclusion. What appeared to be an opportunity was a mirage.

Safety experts, including the author, have urged others to be honest and open about failure. The argument that first stories miss the contributors to failure that closer examination can reveal is surely as true for their own work as for the work of others. The failure of the plan for a research-based approach to patient safety is as object a lesson in how *not* to do safety as surely as is the programmatic approach that was undertaken in 2000. Neither was suited to the problems at hand. Neither produced success.

The Second Story

The monograph *A Tale of Two Stories* sought to contrast the usual first stories that are told of celebrated accidents with the 'second stories' that tell how 'multiple interacting factors in complex systems can combine to produce systemic vulnerabilities to failure ... how the system usually works to manage risks but sometimes fails' (Cook, Woods and Miller, 1998: 2–3).

The intention was to differentiate between the pursuit of a single thread of logic and cause that typifies responses to accidents, and the identification and characterisation of multiple threads of influence and contingency and the cloth that results from the weaving of these threads together. Although accidents were a major factor in generating the critical mass of concern about patient safety, the monograph explicitly disparages them as a 'way in' to the safety problem. Second stories are not descriptions of accidents. Second stories are descriptions of locales in the system where accidents sometimes occur. Developing a second story is difficult because most details of operators' worlds are not easily available and what goes on in the operator's mind is not directly accessible to researchers.

Perhaps the best second story example in the monograph is the blood screening study by Smith et al. (Cook, Woods and Miller, 1998). Smith and his colleagues explored the characteristics of a common blood bank task: screening a sample for antibodies to known, common antigens. The task was performed by technicians and the study was intended to help refine computer-based training tools that might someday be used to train technicians. The study revealed serious flaws in the existing tools used to accomplish the task. Data were entered in a table with many lines and columns making mis-entry likely. Quite different results could be produced by shifting an entry slightly. The problem was one of bookkeeping in a complex ledger rather than one of practitioner knowledge or understanding.

This by-product of the research was important for several reasons. First, it suggested ways that the output from the task could be technically wrong. Second, it indicated the tool that was used to perform the task and showed how that tool was poorly configured for the task. Third, it gave computer-based aid designers a point of departure for the design of both training and a potential computer-based aid to performing the task.

Although there had been accidents involving blood bank tasks, Smith et al. were not trying to address those events or were even motivated by them. Their interest was driven by the need to understand configurations of displays for computer-based systems used in operational environments.

The title *A Tale of Two Stories* was intended to draw a sharp distinction between an accident-driven focus on error and a perspective that sought to explain how systems normally succeed but sometimes fail. The basic tenant of this perspective is that successful and failed operations are derived from the same sources – that the same system that produces the successes is the one that produces the failures. Rather than being qualitatively different from normal operations, accidents are the product of normal operations (Perrow, 1984).

The second story is explicitly grounded in an operator's point of view. It is the story of sharp end work situations and actions. It treats the operator's perspective as privileged. The second story is not a theory or even a model. It is, instead, (1) a deliberately atheoretical view of the work world's complexity, contradictions, and conflicts as they appear to the worker, and (2) a description of the worker's methods, approaches, efforts, and concerns related to these world features. The second story seeks to include the entire range of possible situations that the world can contain rather than just the accident situation. Second stories are attempts to include all the details of the world.

Some have taken 'second story' to refer to a deeper, more nuanced understanding of a particular accident. The need for a more sophisticated, more extensive investigation of accidents is a well-established trope in safety research. Better understanding of accidents might be useful in several ways. But the second story of the monograph is not a better view of an accident but of the system locale in which accidents sometimes occur. *The second story cannot be constructed through the study of accidents alone.*

Resilience and the Second Story

Resilience is a property of systems that confers on them the ability to remain intact and functional despite the presence of threats to their integrity and function. The opposite is brittleness. Resilience aspires to be a theory of systemic function. Whether it can meet the aspiration is unclear. Other chapters in this book address resilience engineering as a theory and resilient health care as a practice.

In contrast to the second story, resilience does not privilege any single perspective. The goal of those who study resilience is to escape the limitations of the operator perspective and understand the system without reference to a single perspective. Resilience theory intends to describe the blunt and sharp ends of the system alike. This systemic view is much more difficult to construct and test than a second story. Doing resilience research is philosophically and technically challenging. Indeed, so far, resilience is better characterised by the few, well worked-out examples than any clear theoretical formulation.

One way of thinking about the relationship between the second story and resilience is that resilience is the integral of the second stories that might be discovered for a system over all the possible perspectives that could be taken.

The Dark Side of Resilience

We are forced to ask whether resilience is a good property of systems. Can resilience have a dark side?

The attraction of resilience engineering has been the prospect of being able to engineer systems that are resistant to disturbances. We want systems to achieve economic success while avoiding catastrophic failure. We want systems that are stable, sustainable, robust, and survive challenges.

Present examples of resilience are ones in which the system performs well in spite of adversity, or sustains itself despite existential threats. We have found these examples because we have looked for them. We have concluded that these examples represent a systemic property because of the similarities we find there.

Hollnagel (2008) has pointed out that accident investigation is of limited value because investigators tend to find what they look for. Accidents in complex systems have so many contributors and hindsight bias is so powerful that the contributors identified are mostly recountings of investigators' pre-existing understandings of how accidents happen. But couldn't the same be said for any investigation of any phenomenon – including resilience?

If resilience is truly a systemic property, it is unlikely to show a strong preference for desirable outcomes. Instead, it is likely that this property produces both good results *and bad ones*. After all, the notions of good and bad are social distinctions, not scientific ones. The paucity of bad results in the catalogue of resilience examples is therefore at once both remarkable and deeply troubling.

Our own, failed attempt to set the patient safety agenda at the beginning of the twenty-first century may be useful here. Was the system that was moving towards critical mass in the 1990s not resilient? The *Tale of Two Stories* monograph challenged the political, social, and intellectual system that ascribed bad outcomes to human error. This challenge was successfully fended off by the socio-political system. The system remained intact and largely undisturbed. Other challenges, notably the quality movement, have met similar fates.

Are such performances not evidence of resilience? Should we not add these examples to the list of resilience cases? And if so, aren't we forced to conclude that resilience may be quite a bad property of systems, at least in some cases? If it is a systemic property, then it must be sometimes undesirable. Mere persistence in the face of disturbance is not, in itself, a good thing.

Patient Safety in the Next Ten Years

The failure of the patient safety program owners to achieve victory in their war on error is now well established. It has been well over a decade since Bill Clinton promised to cut medical errors by 50 per cent in five years. There has been little progress and some might even contend that the situation is presently worse than it was in 2000. In the USA a huge effort to use computers to prevent error has foundered. Strikingly in 2011, well after the money to buy them has been spent, the US Agency for Healthcare Research and Quality (AHRQ) recently sought 'basic research' on how to make computers effective in health care work (AHRQ, 2011). The fact that the need for this research and even a model of how to do it were presented 14 years earlier goes unmentioned.

The programmatic approaches to patient safety appear to be in decline. Early enthusiasm for simulation, team training, checklists, computers, safety culture surveys, and their ilk is either dwindling or gone. As these distractions are exhausted, there may be new opportunities to discover the second stories of system success and failure. If it is itself resilient, resilience may become widely accepted. But the experience from the end of the twentieth century should be a caution to those tempted to embrace resilience. Making progress may require both enhancing resilience and, in some cases, overcoming it.

Chapter 3
Resilience and Safety in Health Care: Marriage or Divorce?

René Amalberti

Introduction

Resilience is a system's ability to adapt to unstable environments (Hollnagel, Woods and Leveson, 2006). Health care is a perfect example of a system that exists in an unstable working environment. The wide variety of patients, geographical settings, socio-professional groups, and medical working conditions make adaptations continuously required; emergencies and accidents are by definition not predictable. The resources are often missing in whole or in part, and the legendary autonomy of professionals is *the* usual solution best to look at patients and situations on a case-by-case basis. For all of these reasons, health care is recognised as being highly adaptable, delivering care in almost any conditions, but often with a great deal of waste. So it is sometimes a question of whether one regards the glass as being half full, or as being half empty.

While the situation is not new, there could even be a need of greater adaptations in the future since health care is rapidly changing, due to the evolution of patients (ageing population, transformation of acute patients into chronic patients), advances of personalised medicine, and rapid discharge protocols associated with non-invasive surgery. More than 20 per cent of citizens in western countries will be over 65 in 2020, with more pathologies, co-morbidities (diabetes, chronic heart failure, asthma, chronic obstructive pulmonary disease [COPD]), needing monitoring (cardiac, renal, diabetes, patients socially isolated) and end-of-life care. The growing volume of patients asking for complicated care is not just a matter of aging, since many of the classic acute pathologies of the 1990s are becoming chronic pathologies of the 2020s (myocardial infarction [MI], cancers, AIDs, renal failure, grafts), with patients living years – and even decades – while their severe diseases are under control.

With such an increase of patients, the medical cost per capita will rapidly increase. This will become totally unaffordable for nations and citizens if the main medical answer remains turning to classic institutions to care for these chronic patients (whether the institutions are hospitals, retirement homes, or rehabilitation centres).

And the problem is even trickier. The length of hospitalisation will continue to decrease for the usual pathologies. Day surgery and day medicine – or at least rapid discharge protocols including deliveries in maternity – will become the norm because of the innovative techniques of care, expected benefits for safety (namely reduction of nosocomial infections), and a drive towards greater cost-effectiveness. Patients will therefore continue to enter home health care (HHC) 'sicker and quicker', often with complex health problems that require extensive intervention (Lang et al., 2009) and with a greater need for adaptation of the medical supply to the specifics of each patient's environment (patient, relatives, facilities, availability of gratuitous and home care aids, etc.). The strategy will predictably move towards a concept of integrated care.

This massive move from hospital to primary and home care will (probably) make the medical system more effective for patients (longer life, healthy life), but also require greater resilience in case-to-case adaptation, hence creating new situations for adverse events. To rephrase, medical effectiveness should benefit from the change (speaking at the national level, with an epidemiological vision). A greater resilience (of workers and organisations) should be a condition of this change, but patient safety (speaking of victims) should not necessarily improve significantly, since the reduced risks from shorter hospital stays will probably be replaced by new types of adverse events.

This is precisely the problem: best safety (lower rate of adverse events), high performance (longer life, healthy life, best money value), and strong resilience (adaptation to the unexpected) do not go together very well. Although there is some evidence in the literature that greater resilience goes well together with greater performance (Amalberti et al., 2006), there is little evidence that being both (ultra) resilient and (ultra) performing on one hand, and (ultra) safe on the other hand is feasible, because of the natural trade-offs that exist between these criteria, especially when the matter comes to the optimisation of one independently of the other (Morel, Amalberti and Chauvin, 2008). The problem is how to trade off total standardisation and supervision (usually needed to optimise safety) against a culture of innovation and personalisation (as opposed to a standardised culture) and a considerable autonomy left to individuals and groups (needed for opportunistic adaptations) (Amalberti et al., 2005).

Most readers will assume that gaining on all dimensions is just a matter of better teamwork, procedures, organisations, and 'must do'. The answer is unfortunately far from being so simple and no industry has been successful in achieving this on the three dimensions at the same time. For example, the ultra-safe aviation and nuclear industries have lost most of their capacity of resilience and are now strenuously trying to recover some. On the other hand, the fishing industry, military aviation in wartime, and, to some extent, the chemical industry, frequently demonstrate a good level of performance and resilience to the multiple surprises occurring in their jobs, although they are not that safe compared to the excellence of aviation or nuclear industries, etc.

Moving the Cursor on the Three Dimensions: Performance, Resilience and Safety: A Tentative Description of the Trading Functions

Four Strategies / Issues in Managing Risks

1. Type A: Everything done in line with recommended protocols: perfect outcome.
2. Type B: Deviations, adaptations to protocol, possibly minor adverse events: perfect outcome despite adverse events.

3. Type C: Cautious strategy waiting for ideal conditions to start: outcome may be affected by delays.
4. Type D: 'Never events' (adverse events that are serious, largely preventable, and of concern to both the public and health care providers for the purpose of public accountability), accident with fatal prognosis or leading to severe permanent harm.

In France, the figures are probably about 40 per cent for Type A, 50 per cent for Type B, 10 per cent for Type C, and 0.1– per cent to 0.5 per cent for Type D. Note that this last figure – one in a 1,000 patients dying or being severely impaired by an adverse event – does not conflict with a total rate of adverse events close to 6.6 per 1,000 days of hospitalisation in France, since the vast majority of these adverse events belong to Case B, harming the patient, but not changing the final prognosis of the cure (Michel et al., 2004).

What about you and your working conditions? How large a percentage is Type B?

Imagine you are a trained rock climber. Your ambition is to climb an impressive rock face in wintry conditions. The job will be done if you are successful in climbing the rock face.

- Case A: you may have achieved success easily, everything going as you expected (weather, rock, fatigue).
- Case B: you may have achieved success in very adverse conditions, overcoming a series of incidents due to the surprisingly unstable nature of the rocks, spending an additional night on the rock face, and possibly suffering from frostbite.
- Case C: conversely, you gave up and postponed the attempt for fear of the foreseen adverse conditions: bad weather, poor personal shape, or any other hindrance.
- Case D: finally, but very rarely, you climbed and suffered from a severe incident, possibly an accident, consequential for your health with an engagement of vital prognostics, such as a fall.

Now transfer this example to medicine; for example, to the case of a 25-year-old patient with testicular cancer.

- Case A: you have delivered ideal care in a big teaching hospital; the healing was total and perfect within a shorter period of time expected by standard protocols.
- Case B: you delivered effective care and cured the patient, despite working in difficult conditions (summertime, chronic staff shortages, local hospital) and despite a succession of minor but true adverse events during the treatment. For example, the central catheter infusion installed by a young locum anaesthesiologist first entered the pleural cavity, and had to be repositioned in an emergency the following day, and later you spent three days after discharge reacting properly to an infection due to poor coordination with primary care. But finally you treated the cancer.
- Case C: considering the understaffing at that time of year in your hospital, and the importance of the best expertise for surgery, you have balanced elements and made the cautious decision to postpone the treatment for three weeks in order to get ideal staffing and expertise conditions to minimise risks of adverse events.
- Case D: the team made an error with a wrong drug dosage, causing a vital threat to the patient spending a month in an intensive care unit (ICU). In addition to the complication, the cancer treatment has been postponed and healing is still not achieved.

Whatever the domain, mountaineering or health care, one will easily agree that Cases A and B are effective, leading to successes, that Case C is safe and careful, but not necessarily effective, and that Case D is unacceptable.

- If the priority is effectiveness and medical performance, we will trust Cases A and B, despite Case B being rather unsafe.
- If the priority is safety, we will trust Cases A and C, despite Case C being moderately effective.
- If the priority is resilience, we will trust Case B as a perfect example and conversely consider Case C as not resilient.
- Only Case D is unacceptable for all users.

Thus the lesson of the example is simple enough: except for obvious errors ('never events') that may worsen and change the final prognosis, all the other cases are acceptable by the medical community in one way or another. Of course, the ideal pattern of care remains the ambition of Case A, but adaptation (Case B) or a cautious strategy (Case C) are even more frequent and considered as acceptable strategies depending on the local context, and the patients' and professionals' preferences and culture.

Having said that, the health care system is also chronically a bit schizophrenic or even utopian, trying at the same time to adopt an industrial schema of stable and rigid organisation, with increasingly standardised protocols (Øvretveit and Klazinga, 2008), and to adopt technical and organisational innovations, change protocols (half-life of protocols is 5.5 years in many medical specialities (cf. Sjohania et al., 2007), and work with unstable conditions (staff shortages, etc.).

Part of these ambiguities comes from the confusions existing on the definitions, means and ends related to the concepts of medical performance, patient safety and resilience.

Chasing Ambiguities to Adopt a System Vision

Ambiguity of Definition, Means and Ends Related to Medical Performance

The advent of quality and safety (Q&S) in health care has been beneficial but has led to confusion about the ultimate goal of health care.

Nations have for centuries aimed to give their citizens a longer and healthier life. The continuous progresses in medicine, combined with the economic growth of countries, have increased human life expectancy during the past two decades at the incredible rate of three months per year on average.

Although Q&S efforts are important for many crucial aspects (victims, money value), they have probably contributed little to this incredible improvement. The Q&S approach has demonstrated the potential to optimise the value of existing strategies and organisations by a factor of two or three at best, while adopting other innovations may improve the outcome on life expectancy by a factor 10 or even more. For example, anesthesia-related mortality has decreased about 10-fold over the past 20 years. The consensus is that the greatest safety gains have arisen from the introduction of new drugs and techniques in the 1980s and 1990s (propofol, upper airways monitoring and assistance systems, etc.). Better compliance with safeguards and rules accounted for only a limited fraction of these gains. Similarly, survival after liver transplantation has improved from about 10 per cent at one year in the 1960s to over 70 per cent at five years today. The introduction of ciclosporin in the early 1980s alone has increased one-year graft survival from 10 per cent to 55 per cent (Degos et al., 2009).

It is therefore obvious that medical innovation will continue to be the leading factor for professionals and patients maintaining hope in better medical issues. The half-life of knowledge in medicine is assumed to be around five years. But there are signs that obsolescence may occur within two years for 23 per cent of the most valuable reviews of literature, and within one year for 15 per cent.

Quality and safety will be sacrificed any time an innovation is in competition (Sjohania et al., 2007).

To rephrase, the ultimate goal and judgement for performance will be the outcome and not the process. Should the patient be cured or their life significantly extended with healthy conditions, the result will be considered much better than any strategy advocating no default, no error, or total compliance to the recommended procedures and organisations, but in the end, a shorter life.

Ambiguity of Means and Ends Related to Patient Safety

Patient safety is usually defined as the absence of harm to patient. The number of errors and adverse events (AEs) counted in National Adverse Events Studies is considerable. Almost 10 per cent of hospital patients experience an adverse event and about 40 per cent of events are preventable. This is true for all Western countries (Baker et al., 2004).

Unfortunately, the error rate is growing than reducing, thanks to a set of naïve visions of risk management in medicine (Vincent et al., 2008). Due to innovation, we continuously change strategies, so that what was the recommended strategy last year may be an error this year. By multiplying process-driven solutions, we create space for non-compliance that invariably results in more errors (Carthey et al., 2011). The safer we make the system, the more we look for less important events; we are not clear on the distinction between near misses and misses, and therefore we count events that are near misses as misses. We increase the complexity of care patterns and organisations, resulting in more interfaces and communication problems. Last but not least, lawyers have progressively expanded the vision of adverse events to get money, tentatively blaming any imperfect care when the pathology is severe with a bad outcome, regardless of whether or not this imperfect care has contributed really to harm the patient (typical of case mix).

One will easily agree that there is no hope in seeing the total of AEs going down in the future with such a naïve, unstable and interpretative approach of safety.

We need to revise means and ends. Patient safety should widen its vision and become more system-oriented.

We should never forget that only one in 1,000 AEs leads to death and, although the calculation is scarcely made, that very few AEs change the prognosis of the treatment. Let us consider, for example, an infusion line of chemotherapy going outside a vein in the arm. It will cause a severe lymphangitis, requiring weeks to recover. No doubt that it is an AE. However, the patient suffering this AE will probably be cured of their cancer at the end of the care process, hence this AE will not be contradictory to a count of global improvement, longer life duration, and healthy life. It seems obvious that patient safety should widen the narrow timeframe used in AE detection and analysis and make a clear distinction between what is important to health care (longer life, healthy life) and what is important to a justice and insurance-driven approach searching for compensation and money for all errors / non-compliance, whatever the consequence of the prognosis (Amalberti et al., 2011).

The ultimate goal of patient safety should, therefore, move to avoid any problem that may worsen the final prognosis of the pathology, the patient's length of life, and the conditions of life (quality of healthy life). But to adopt such a healing-oriented definition, the strategies of patient safety and quality would have to change significantly.

Ambiguity of Means and Ends Related to Resilience (in Health Care)

Medicine is known to be a land of adaptation and sometimes improvisation, whether those adaptations and improvisations are justified or not.

The results of patients' outcomes of such a high level of non-compliance to recommended procedures are disputed. Quality and safety officers, together with lawyers, see this attitude as an evil, advocating, for example, that only 55 per cent of surgical patients receive antimicrobial prophylaxis (Bratzler et al., 2005) and only 58 per cent of those at risk of venous thromboembolism receive the recommended preventive treatment (Cohen et al., 2008). However, other professionals tend to disagree and justify the adjustments as needed. For example, a peer-review panel judged medical exceptions to 16 chronic disease and prevention quality measures as appropriate, inappropriate, or of uncertain appropriateness. The frequency of inappropriate medical exceptions to quality measures appeared to be incredibly high, although they were considered by these peers to be correct most of the time (Persell et al., 2011).

The truth is probably in between these two extreme positions. There is no justification to disregard recommended protocol when the context and conditions make the protocol applicable, except when the chosen solution is proven to be worse for the medical outcome. This is probably the case for half of the patients. On the other hand, there are billions of situations where we do not have recommended protocols, either because none exist, or more frequently, because they have been established out of the context of co-morbidities and working conditions of the current patient setting. This contrast requires redefining what we expect from greater resilience in health care.

If resilience is seen as the capacity to adapt to unexpected and unstable environments, it undoubtedly appears to be an ecological and natural quality of health care. It is therefore not a priority to increase resilience in health care. The ultimate priority is probably to maintain natural resilience for difficult situations, and abandon some for the standard.

On the other hand, resilience is not a (good) solution for coping with non-compliance, taking useless risks by negligence, and then managing the risk afterwards, thanks to a supposed ability in resilience. Resilience is only required when the standard solution cannot apply, although this case may represent a large number of cases.

Note also that this discussion of resilience is totally different from the discussion of resilience in aviation or the nuclear industry, where the very problem is to reinject resilience that has disappeared or been sacrificed for the benefit of a fully rigid supervised and standardised system.

Conclusion

Performance, safety, and resilience have developed in a silo vision of health care during the last decades. The problems that this causes have not been perceived, since the developments in each dimension were in their infancy. The situation is worsening because of the progresses made in each dimension and the natural tendency to optimise each one independently of the other.

Most of the ambiguities in means and ends of performance, resilience and safety remained invisible for a long time or were at least not considered problematic. But now they are. We need to revisit the concepts, to give better definition, to adopt a system perspective and apply the art of compromise.

The growth in medical performance will undoubtedly continue with the emphasis on innovation, but also accepting that quality approaches are necessary to get the expected benefits of innovation fully. Safety will improve only if we abandon the naïve vision imposed on health care for years when counting adverse events and adopt a widened timeframe for considering and judging problems. Last, a growth of resilience is not by itself the solution for improving health care performance and safety, since the level of resilience is already probably too high. The best solution should rather consist in applying even more resilience to the numerous cases generated by the complexity and the variety of the medical system, but at the same time, less resilience to the standard cases. Adopting a system perspective and global vision may serve to balance the three dimensions, with the unique ultimate goal of providing more citizens with longer and healthier lives. All other goals are artificial, disputable, and subject to local drawbacks (Amalberti, 2013).

Chapter 4
What Safety-II Might Learn from the Socio-cultural Critique of Safety-I

Justin Waring

Introduction

First we should praise the significant advances that have been made in the area of patient safety. This includes the dedication and energy of individuals and groups who have made safety a pre-eminent health policy issue and worked to change the way we think about safety, devising innovative methods for safety research and developing interventions, technologies and guidelines that promote safer working and more robust learning (Waring et al., 2010).

That said, patient safety remains a very real and significant problem; first, for patients in terms of unanticipated suffering, prolonged care and in some cases unexpected death, but also for service leaders in terms of how best to improve the quality and safety of their services. It might even be argued that despite the advances in theory and research, there has been little evidence of sustained safety improvement (Landrigan et al., 2010). We might argue, therefore, that we need to reflect more thoroughly on how we think about the 'problem' of patient safety itself. Much of the emphasis to date has been on changing how we think about the sources of 'unsafe' care within complex organisations (e.g. Kohn, Corrigan and Donaldson, 2000; Department of Health, 2000), whilst giving little consideration to what makes care 'safe'. Despite leaders in safety science highlighting both the positive and negative aspects of safety (Hollnagel, Woods and Leveson, 2006; Reason, 1997), it seems that the negative dimension has garnered greater interest. As such, strategies and interventions have typically been directed at eradicating risk, rather than promoting resilience. It is arguably unfair to be critical of a movement that ostensibly seeks to improve patient health and well-being, but if we are to progress the safety of our healthcare systems, perhaps we need to think more critically about the nature of the problem itself, or at least how it has been framed in mainstream approaches. The shift from Safety-I to Safety-II highlights how new lines of thinking can offer additional possibilities for safety improvement that build on, rather than replace, recent advances through taking a more proactive and less reactive approach. The aim of this chapter is to highlight some of the sociocultural critiques of the Safety-I approach, and to think how future advances in Safety-II might avoid similar dilemmas.

After establishing that clinical errors, mishaps and risks were a significant issue (e.g. Brennan et al., 1991), the challenge facing policy-makers and scholars of the mid-1990s was how to explain why these events came about and how they might be prevented. At this time, it remained difficult for many professional communities, and indeed political and public groups, to come to terms with the scale and significance of iatrogenic disease (see also Illich, 1976). It was still the view that lone risk-takers or bad apples were the problem and little explicit account was taken of the inherent uncertainties and risks to clinical practice (Fox, 1980).

At this juncture, we see the coming together of two influential lines of thought. The first involved a fundamental reconceptualisation of 'human error' from theories and concepts developed largely in social psychology, ergonomics and human factors (Rasmussen and Jensen, 1974; Reason, 1997; Vincent, 1993). The second was to find ways of reducing risk by drawing on the lessons of what are often called high reliability organisations (HROs), such as those practices found in aviation, petrochemicals and nuclear energy (Roberts, 1990; Rochlin et al., 1987; Schulman, 1993; Weick, 1987) that have since been applied in the health care context (Provonost et al., 2006; Roberts, 1990; Thomas et al., 2004). With regards to the first, Safety-I is commonly associated with the idea that 'active' human errors are often enabled, exacerbated or conditioned by 'latent' factors located within the wider organisation of work. As such, efforts to improve safety should not look solely at individual wrongdoing and blame, but instead at the influence of systemic factors. With regards to the second, Safety-I usually involves the creation of procedures that enable learning about safety events through identifying actual or potential instances of unsafe practice and then locating the relevant upstream factors that should be controlled to prevent reoccurrence (Reason, 1997). This often entails some form of risk management system to capture and analyse safety reports, the creation of a safety culture that encourages staff awareness, mindfulness of safety, openness and communication; and the implementation of strategies that reduce the risk of human error through standardisation, simplification and checking. Clearly, this short summary does little justice to the enormous advances made in the theory and practice, but it highlights some of the features of what is sometimes characterised as the 'measure and manage' orthodoxy of patient safety (Rowley and Waring, 2011).

Critical Analysis of Patient Safety-I

The first line of critique resonates strongly with the Safety-II approach and the work of Hollnagel and colleagues (e.g. Hollnagel, Woods and Leveson, 2006). That is, the mainstream approach is based upon a highly technocratic and largely retrospective model of learning. In short, safety breaches are to be identified, analysed and then their antecedents controlled. First and foremost, this involves learning from and rectifying *the past* without necessarily thinking about more proactive forms of foresight and problem-solving (see Chapter 1 for a more thorough discussion). Linked to this, it focuses its efforts on the 10–20 per cent of reported safety breaches (which is relatively common to healthcare organisation, although not necessarily other complex settings), rather than the 80–90 per cent of instances that maintain day-to-day safety. In line with the work of Mesman (2011), it misses the huge opportunities for learning found in the hidden resources and resilience of day-to-day safe clinical practice. Where more proactive techniques have been used, such as failure mode and effect analysis or prospective hazard analysis techniques, they tend to emphasise the sources of risk, without necessarily trying to focus on the more diverse sources of safety, and replicate a managerial or technocratic approach to learning and change.

More than this, however, the model of systems thinking and 'root cause' analysis that informs Safety-I too often focuses on what might be considered the clinical micro-system, rather than the wider sociocultural, organisational system or wider political environment (Waring, 2007a). In other words, it often focuses on how communication, team work, resource management, or workload planning interfere with safe operations, and not the influence of inter-departmental processes, cultures and identities, management practices, or political decision-making. Where attention is paid to this level, we find that the organisation of health care is often so complex, non-linear and tightly-coupled that the idea of creating a reliable, standardised and safe system remains a 'wicked problem' (Rittel and Webber, 1973 ; Waring, McDonald and Harrison, 2006; Waring, Harrison and McDonald, 2007).

The second line of criticism relates to the reliance upon retrospective learning and risk management systems. Arguably, the most common problem relates to staff communication or reporting, which continues to be inhibited by organisational, professional and cultural barriers (Braithwaite, Hyde and Pope, 2010; Waring, 2005). We should not overlook the enormous organisational demands of undertaking detailed incident reviews and building reports for consumption by multiple audiences and stakeholders (Braithwaite et al., 2006; Nicolini et al., 2011). More significantly, there is little proof that the type of evidence developed through these activities aligns with the knowledge and skills of front-line clinicians. Research on the investigation of safety events shows their limited scope for engendering learning and change, often because they are caught between the demands of public accountability and bureaucratic process, whilst the outcomes of inquiries are typically in the forms of documented recommendations or prescriptive procedures that are not easily translated and implemented into practice (Nicolini et al., 2011). In short, there is often a gap between those on the front line and those who 'manage' safety. This is evidenced by the limited number of safety events that are communicated 'upwards' or outside front-line clinical communities and the difficulties of service leaders to implement 'downward' changes in established clinical practices.

The Sociocultural Dilemmas for Patient Safety

Drawing particularly on the work of Douglas (1994), three underlying sociocultural dilemmas characterise the prevailing approach to patient safety. The first relates to the issue of epistemology and knowledge. For the most part, the orthodox approach sees safety events or risks as inherently 'real' and tangible, about which objective knowledge or evidence can be established. A major ambition of the movement has been to establish common definitions, taxonomies or typologies through which safety events can be better identified and classified (Chang et al., 2005; Donaldson, 2009). Moreover, various approaches and tools are used to assess, stratify and sort risk, such as risk matrices or fish-bone templates (Woloshynowych et al., 2005). It is through better classification, identification and analysis that learning is to occur. However, this 'techno-scientific' approach struggles to recognise that knowledge about safety is also *constructed* within particular epistemic and cultural communities, such as those of professional or clinical groups.

Social constructionism is a philosophical approach to the nature of knowledge that suggests knowledge about the world is not objective in the form of independent 'facts' or 'evidence', but rather it is produced through subjective interaction, shared social conventions and prevailing beliefs (Hacking, 1999; Gergen, 2009). This means that *all* the ways we see, make sense of and giving meaning to the world are shaped by prevailing languages, cultures and social processes, including scientific enquiries (Knorr-Cetina, 1981). This perspective therefore questions the status of knowledge and suggests that, whilst there may indeed be a 'real world' or ontology, the only way we can understand and give meaning to this in time is through social and cultural processes. Beyond this rather basic description, there remains considerable debate about social constructionism, especially the extent to which all 'things' can be viewed as socially constructed and the implicit role of moral and ideology judgement often found within constructionist accounts (Hacking, 1999).

For our purposes here, a social constructionist perspective highlights for us the idea that what one group may see as a threat to safety, or indeed, source of resilience, may not be seen in the same way by another group. In one sense, we might therefore think of safety knowledge as 'slippery' in order to reflect the difficulty of establishing one agreed definition. This is important, because how we understand the problem of safety is inherently linked to how we seek to solve it. Another issue relates to the idea that knowledge is also 'sticky'; that is, it is deeply embedded within, and not easily de-coupled from, closely connected groups of social actors, or professional silos, and is therefore difficult to share with or communicate to outside groups (Szulanski, 2003). This is especially relevant to the problems of knowledge sharing, incident reporting and the spread of safety innovations (Waring, 2005). The processes of sense-making has been shown as being integral to organisational reliability and resilience (Weick, 1995), but it remains important to remember that the way people make sense of what is safe or unsafe is framed by the prevailing and divided cultural norms and values. So, greater attention to the complexity of knowledge, or how people interpret events within a cultural context, is essential to any model of learning and improvement.

The second dilemma relates to the issue of culture. The idea of a 'safety culture' is prominent in reliability and safety research for demonstrating the importance of collective sense-making, mindfulness to danger, communication and taking a proactive approach to risk (e.g. Flin, 2007; Guldenmund, 2000). This is often seen as a counterpoint to a 'blame culture', as it encourages clinicians to recognise appropriately the latent sources of risk, to report their experiences and to participate in change programmes. Illustrating the 'measure and manage' orthodoxy, there remains considerable interest in using surveys and tools to determine the extent to which an organisation or department possess a 'safe' culture (e.g. AHRQ Survey of Patient Safety Culture, Manchester Patient Safety Framework). Without engaging in long-rehearsed debates about whether cultures can appropriately be measured as espoused attitudes, it is arguably the case that the idea of a 'safety', or even 'blame', culture is something of a conceptual shorthand. Cultures cannot be allocated into discrete categories or along descriptive spectra, but remain highly complex elements of social life that reflect the underlying cognitive, normative and moral frameworks that structure distinct social groups. Despite its importance for the social sciences, 'culture' remains a surprisingly complex and ambiguous concept. It is often held that cultures are composed of different levels, from more visible artefacts to more deeply-held beliefs (Schein, 2004). Equally, cultures are sometimes seen as having a 'structuring' and (dys) functional effect on group behaviours and performance, whereas others see cultures as being emergent from social interaction and sites for both inter- and intra-group conflict (Parker, 2000). Conceptualising cultures as safer or less safe can overlook the influence of various aspects of cultures within their wider social context, such as the complex links between attitudes towards safety, identity and professionalism. As research shows, learning to cope with risk is often seen as a hallmark of professionalism, rather than a trait of an unsafe culture (Waring et al., 2007).

Building on the above, cultures also have an important political dimension. On the one hand, shared norms and moral codes provide a basis of social order 'within' communities through binding people together and guiding expected social behaviours, especially in response to issues of risk (Douglas, 1994). How one social group responds to what is seen as a risk might differ from another, as evidenced by variations in incident reporting. On the other hand, they also provide a basis of social order between communities, through a shared sense of belonging and inter-group differentiation. The issue of risk again becomes important in this process, through binding people together in their understandings and opposition to risky behaviours (Douglas, 1994). In other words, creating or fostering a safety culture is not only difficult but needs to navigate the different cultural topographies that characterise a highly skilled and professionalised workforce.

The third dilemma relates to the issue of power. Building on the above, the cultural framing of risk is closely linked to the politics of blame (Douglas, 1994). Taking a sociocultural perspective, we can see that practically all understandings of risk, and with them preferences for how risks should be controlled, function as strategies to allocate responsibility. This is widely recognised in the safety literature, but it is usually associated with a person-centred understanding of risk that fails to recognise upstream factors (Reason, 1997). Although a systems approach might appear to move away from blaming those on the front line, it still involves some process of allocating responsibility. Arguably, all risk management systems aim to identify and control for the sources of risk and, as such, they represent a powerful medium for controlling social behaviours or communities that are deemed to be risky (Douglas, 1994).

Returning to the point discussed above, the 'techno-scientific' approach is typically presented as objective, scientific and neutral, and therefore beyond the politics of risk. Yet arguably, it still functions to allocate responsibility and blame. When these systems are located within complex political environments, such as health care, they become prominent tools of social order through categorising and control 'risky' or 'at risk' practices (Waring, 2010). For example, patient safety reporting systems, together with similar instances of quality assurance and clinical governance, have been interpreted as complex mechanisms of organisation control over the indeterminate and 'hard to reach' aspects of professional practice (Waring, 2007b). Equally, cultures can come into conflict and resist dominant ideas, especially where they threaten the shared values and sense of community that binds people together. As such, the promotion of safety and risk can become prominent 'flash points' in the disputes between occupational and organisational groups.

Drawing together these three dilemmas, we might argue that the prevailing approach to patient safety struggles to accommodate different ways of thinking about safety, to appreciate that cultures are very difficult to change and that issues of power are often inherent to complex professionalised work places. The role of professions and professionalism are particularly central to this approach. These experts, usually in privileged occupations, represent highly developed 'epistemic communities' that have deeply held ways of making sense and giving meaning to their work (Knorr-Cetina, 1981). Moreover, they are bound together by shared norms, beliefs and identities that are acquired through training and socialisation and shape day-to-day practice (Lave and Wenger, 1991). By virtue of their expertise and contributions to society, professionals represent influential groups that are often accorded a high degree of discretion in their work but also influence others (Freidson, 1970). Health care professionals exhibit well established ways of dealing with unsafe or risky performance that reflect their shared knowledge and culture and tend to reinforce their status or reputation (Freidson, 1970; Rosenthal, 1995). This is an important observation because new ways of managing quality or safety typically interact with these established procedures and compete to introduce new ways of defining the problem, change cultures and impose new lines of authority (Pollitt, 1990; Waring, 2007b). As such, they might be seen as working against, rather than with, professional communities – hence the problems of implementation. In the future, we may need to look at how safety improvements work *with* and *within* professional communities where possible.

Summary

The dilemmas outlined in this chapter could equally apply to more proactive approaches to safety. As such, there is much that Patient Safety-II can learn from the sociocultural critique of Patient Safety-II. In particular, we need to consider that 'safety' and being 'safe' can mean different things to different groups; that communities and groups will place different values and norms on 'what makes things safe' and why they should change their behaviours, and that Safety-II will also play into long-standing political faultlines that characterise modern health care, especially those between doctors, nurses and managers.

We need to find ways of establishing a common terminology and shared referential framework that enables clinicians from different backgrounds to talk about and agree upon what produces safety. We need to find methods of bringing together clinicians in ways that recognise and, in most instances, respect, or at least work with, different values and beliefs so as to foster integration and mutuality as the basis of shared practices. And we need to think about how intractable differences, especially power disputes, can be reconciled to ensure that the safety of patients is put ahead of sectional interests. If we want to build more adaptive, resilient and, ultimately safer health care systems, we should therefore think more critically about the assumptions that guide our thinking, especially as they relate to questions of knowledge, culture and power.

Key Points

How we understand the problem of patient safety is inherently linked to how we seek to solve it.

- It is difficult to establish single and commonly agreed definitions of error, risk or safety because social groups have different ways of making sense of these issues.
- It is difficult to change cultures because they are deeply ingrained within both day-to-day social practice and tied to wider social conditions.
- It is important to recognise the dynamics of power in complex social organisations and how issues of control and competition are integral to thinking about risks and their control.
- Professional communities represent strong groups bound together by shared knowledge and cultures and represent powerful organisational actors. Attempts to change how we manage the quality and safety of these groups are particularly difficult.

Chapter 5
Looking at Success versus Looking at Failure: Is Quality Safety? Is Safety Quality?

Sam Sheps and Karen Cardiff

Introduction

Advocates of resilience engineering highlight, and increasingly emphasise, examining success rather than focusing solely on failure: why things go right rather than why they go wrong (Hollnagel et al., 2006; Woods, 2003; Woods and Branlat, 2011a). It is thought that more can be learned from how processes go right most of the time, rather than spending inordinate time and effort on examining things that go wrong. However, given that the notion of success in health care has a long history of being portrayed primarily in terms of quality, we are concerned that health care will at best be divided on what the message from resilience engineering means, or more likely, will miss the point entirely. Instead of seizing an opportunity to pay attention to, and reflect on, the nature of success in complex adaptive systems, it is relatively easy to imagine that health care's default reaction will be to link success with activities designed to improve quality. This chapter explains why this might happen and why we should care.

The heart of the matter is that health care does not make a clear distinction between quality and safety (Cardiff, 2007; Dekker, 2007; Resar, 2007; Vincent, 2010). It is fuzzy at best, since safety is often viewed as one of a number of attributes of quality that also include access, 'best practices' in diagnosis, treatment and follow-up, patient satisfaction and/or efficiency. This conflation of quality and safety is problematic for a number of reasons. In practical terms, conflating the concepts can result in investing efforts in solving the wrong problem and potentially misappropriates limited human and financial resources. For example, most of the current approaches to safety are focused on activities designed to improve the quality of care (Institute for Healthcare Improvement, 2012), rather than preparing frontline staff to cope with the complexity that they face on a daily basis, as well as the unexpected nature of adverse events (Bagian, 2007). We see a shift in emphasis from failure to success (as a source of learning) as potentially, if inadvertently, reinforcing the conflation of quality and safety, since it is not difficult to predict that success will continue to be credited by many in health care to ongoing quality initiatives. With success disguised as an outcome of quality efforts, the benefits and value of examining success as an emergent feature of complex adaptive systems will not be realised.

In no other risk-critical industry are quality and safety so conflated. This is the case not because these industries have no metrics for quality or safety, but rather because they experience – and thus view them – as two quite distinct organisational challenges, thus requiring quite different approaches in order to be achieved. Not so in health care, where quality is based on the assumption that problems can be fixed and improvement requires an assessment of what the problem is, that, in turn, leads to a specific solution. It is a 'diagnosis and treat' ethos deeply embedded within all health care activities. Patient safety generally follows the same logic: critical incidents are investigated (retrospectively and often superficially), problems are identified, and recommendations made (DX / RX). The discourse on safety in health care is thus unlike the discourse about safety in other risk-critical industries. Vincent (2010) points out that there are also important social differences between the people who consider themselves quality advocates and those who consider themselves safety advocates.

Because of the conflation of safety with quality, safety is seen as an attribute of quality (a goal to be reached and maintained e.g., the elimination of 'never events', and achievement of a stable 'error-free' state) rather than an emergent, thus dynamic, property of everyday work to manage trade-offs without doing harm. This perspective also tends to reinforce the notion that critical events are linear, thus easily described, despite the reality that every event has a 'first story' (simple and linear) and a 'second story' that reveals the complex dynamics involved (Cook, Woods and Miller, 1998; Dekker, 2006a; Dekker, Cilliers and Hofmeyr, 2011). Thus health care does a poor job of understanding sources of failure in the complex adaptive system it represents.

However, until health care begins to examine the broader social and organisational contexts within which safe care (and critical incidents) arise, the conflation of quality and safety won't go away (Rowley and Waring, 2011). Moreover, the wisdom and insight of experts such as Perrow (1999), Rochlin (1999), Rasmussen (1997), Weick (1998), Hollnagel (2009a), and Cook and Woods (1994) regarding everyday work in complex adaptive systems will continue to be misunderstood, misquoted, underestimated or largely ignored.

In health care, quality, at least rhetorically, is not seen to be related in any way to trade-offs in everyday work: indeed the primacy and logic of the quality agenda is that it should never be traded off for other ends – e.g., cost – and thus dismisses the reality of goal conflicts or trade-offs in everyday work (Woods and Branlat, 2011b; Hoffman and Woods, 2011). Moreover, the achievement of quality is largely perceived as the control of variability through administrative and clinical procedures, guidelines, rules and education, e.g., the competencies movement (National Health Service, 2012; Shaw, Jelfs and Franklin, 2012). More recently, quality has been bound tightly to efficiency, specifically getting rid of 'waste' (itself superficially believed to be a bad thing) through a heavy emphasis on Lean thinking (Narusawa and Shook, 2009). It does not lend itself to addressing the dynamic nature of health care provision, but seeks to dampen the dynamic nature of health care by generating rules (e.g., right person, right time, right drug), thus ignoring the need to address goal conflicts (e.g., 'faster-better-cheaper', distributing versus concentrating autonomy, responsibility and authority, efficiency-thoroughness) (Hollnagel, 2009a; Hoffman and Woods, 2011; Cook, 2012).

Indeed, quality is pursued as a state of excellence (often unfortunately referred to as 'best practices') to be attained (and maintained) and does not admit the necessity of addressing itself to organisational adaptive capacity in the face of surprises (unexpected) or reasonably well-known challenges (more or less expected): these issues, it is believed, will take care of themselves when high quality is achieved. However, Hoffman and Woods (2011) argue that 'optimizing over some demands leads to brittleness when encountering other demands'. For example, the contribution of adaptation of work through resilience to meet the surprises of everyday work is the antithesis of quality, which works through benchmarks of what are considered 'best practices', and thus adaptation is likely to be underappreciated and or mistaken for inefficiency.

Safety thinking, on the other hand, must acknowledge both expected and unexpected variation in work. It seeks to articulate and understand this reality so that the dynamic nature of work can be managed appropriately and the inherent trade-offs acknowledged and understood in order to keep the system within a safe operating space (Hollnagel, 2009a). Quality represents, as it is understood in health care, a set of non-dynamic attributes of the daily work of both providers and organisations. This creates problems at the governance level, where this view is most strongly held, and where it becomes an important and limiting aspect of organisational culture. Interestingly at the sharp end of care, reality to some extent has engendered the perception of the essentially dynamic nature of care and the necessity of trade-offs, although perhaps not to the point of accepting 'accidents' as normal (Perrow, 1999).

The blunt end sees 'accidents' as lapses in performance due to inadequate education regarding clinical processes or basic knowledge and thus engenders a deeply felt sense of personal / professional inadequacy in a context in which trade-offs (performance pressures) are strongly felt, but only incompletely understood. The quality agenda and professional self-esteem thus subtly emphasise the notion of personal competence, obscuring the system issues influencing (and often creating problems in) daily work. Unfortunately, the revival of personal competency (as the cornerstone of accountability) as a major theme became particularly apparent to us while attending the 2010 Patient Safety Congress in Birmingham. In addition, the blunt end also tends to focus on the failure to follow procedures and policies as a 'root cause' of adverse events as a result of performance variation, which must be controlled (Cook and Nemeth, 2010). This approach generally leads to more policies and procedures that serve only to compound the already complex nature of care by increasing the number of trade-offs required to do normal work (Grote, 2006) but they persist, since they primarily serve important purposes for organisations and their leaders (Dekker, Nyce and Myers, 2012; Cook and Nemeth, 2010).

The quality agenda in health care is also essentially reactive. It seeks to fix problems after they occur rather than trying to anticipate and build defensive mechanisms prospectively. This retrospective approach immediately and inadvertently injects hindsight bias into the investigative process that in turn leads to less, rather than more, learning (Dekker, 2006a). It is a reductionist process that does not / cannot fully comprehend the complex dynamics, intrinsic to the work itself, which can create critical incidents. In addition, it leads to trivial, if not completely useless, recommendations that tend to focus on competency issues (education) or lack of procedural adherence (more rules), both designed to fix a highly specific set of circumstances.

Moreover, wider system trade-offs and the capacity to respond are not generally addressed ('the organisation is fine, but the people need to be fixed or occasionally the rules updated'). Ironically, more rules or training to comply often have the effect of making both care processes and the organisation generally more brittle, less adaptable and therefore less safe. Interestingly, recent risk management literature has observed that education often has the effect of creating worse outcomes (Card, Ward and Clarkson, 2012), not to mention its potential to degrade staff morale.

The quality agenda also includes – sometimes solely consists of – the problem of inefficiencies (waste or valueless activities) without sufficient consideration for, or by, whom waste or value is defined. Since the health care system is designed, primarily, to meet the needs of providers (and only incidentally meets the needs of patients) the quality agenda, while said to be patient-centered, rarely actually is. Looking for waste (activities without value) is largely an organisational initiative to enhance efficiency; that is, to save money. However, this approach, if applied to non-linear clinical processes, can inadvertently reduce the capacity of the organisation (broadly and locally) to respond to challenges, since that capacity is rarely taken into account (Cook, 2012).

The conflation of safety with quality assumes that improving quality will address safety issues. This assumption is largely untrue and can have the baleful influence of setting up organisations, and the people who work in them, for a hard emotional fall when critical incidents occur.

Returning to the issue of what success means in relation to quality, if it is defined as the ability of the organisation to maintain functioning in the face of challenges, rather than as a normative value of excellence, there should be no problem with looking at success (i.e. Safety-II) to foster a safer operating environment. However, if quality has normative characteristics / value, as outlined above (and which we believe largely to be the case), then health care will see success and quality as equivalent and, as it has in the past, will continue misdirecting its efforts to enhance safety. Moreover, health care will fail to understand the key attributes of resilience and thus will fail to monitor its organisational and clinical activities closely (especially trade-offs), to anticipate the unexpected, especially the truly surprising (Wears and Webb, 2011), to understand the need for and capacity to respond to events when they arise and thus (more generally) to learn.

What's to be Done?

A relatively new conceptualisation that will both allow us to focus on success and avoid falling into the trap that success simply means quality is the elaboration of Safety-I and Safety-II (Chapter 1). Hollnagel has defined Safety-I as the focus on adverse events and, through investigation, attempts to reduce their number. As described above, this is the dominant posture of most health care organisations with regard to safety and risk management. Safety-II, on the other hand, is defined as attending to everyday work, why it succeeds and how to foster that success, thus putting an emphasis on understanding the resilience of the system by providing a deeper understanding of the ways in which challenges to operations are anticipated and met.

As noted above, this directs our attention to four key capabilities: *to respond* to every day work and unexpected events as they arise; *to monitor* and understand current work processes; *to learn* from past experience; and *to anticipate* those challenges in order to prevent or mitigate their effects. Developing these capabilities takes us considerably further along the road to a greater understanding of how to enhance patient safety, and avoids getting us entangled in the quality / safety confusion. Safety-II does not ignore the basic rules, policies, procedures and competencies that provide the bedrock for normal and successful practice (and that fall within the rubric of Safety-I), but it moves us away from seeing safety only in terms of these considerations. It engages us to think much more deeply about how everyday work gets done (as opposed to how we imagine it gets done), how and why actors in complex dynamic systems do what they do (mostly well), and what we can learn about that success to foster a greater capacity for maintaining it, while looking ahead to understanding the many things (expected and unexpected) that might be a challenge to successful operations.

The current preoccupation with failure, whether in safety or quality terms, prevents our gaining a broader and more dynamic perspective needed to enhance safety. Indeed, the recent paper by Landrigan et al. (2010) demonstrating that the rates of critical incidents (in ten North Carolina hospitals said to be at the forefront of the patient safety movement) remained essentially the same in the decade following the Institute of Medicine Report *To Err is Human* (Kohn, Corrigan and Donaldson, 2000) should demand our attention. The established concepts of resilience engineering and their emerging application in health care as Safety-II thinking can assist us in overcoming the impasse highlighted by Landrigan et al. (2010). In particular, and in contrast to most quality improvement strategies, Safety-II recognises that dynamic work settings require a flexible approach to everyday work. Performance variation is both necessary and useful. This is what helps create success.

However, this is an antithesis to the thinking of a currently very popular and well publicised (Kenney, 2010; Institute for

Healthcare Improvement, 2012; Wellman, Jeffries and Hagan, 2011; *The New York Times*, 2010) quality improvement strategy such as Lean (Narusawa and Shook, 2009) that emphasises (often very prescriptively) the standardisation of work processes and where staff are encouraged to imagine a system with no variation in work or practice. Indeed, problems arise when this 'one size fits all' approach is applied to complex human organisations (Solow and Fake, 2010). Lean (Narusawa and Shook, 2009), like the classic quality model, creates the illusion that safety, once established, can be maintained by keeping the performance of the system's parts (human and technical) within certain bounds (e.g., people should not violate rules and procedures). The goal is to keep performance variability under control. This mantra seriously limits the capacity of an organisation to respond to the unexpected, and thus prevent or mitigate harm. We must, therefore, be vigilant and not allow Safety-II to be hijacked by quality improvement gurus and taken simply as a reformulation of the quality agenda. That clearly is not the way forward for patient safety.

Chapter 6
Health Care as a Complex Adaptive System

Jeffrey Braithwaite, Robyn Clay-Williams, Peter Nugus and Jennifer Plumb

Introduction

This chapter frames resilience in the context of health care as a complex adaptive system (CAS). We initially introduce relevant systems concepts, and then discuss health care as a CAS, presenting and analysing three case studies illuminating key characteristics. Then we discuss resilience in the health care CAS.

Characterising Systems

A system is a collection of components (for example, cells, people or technological devices) that cohere in a pattern or structure to produce a function or outcome (Meadows, Meadows and Randers, 1992). Systems are circumscribed by their boundaries, and can be to a greater or lesser extent closed or open. These perimeters can range from somewhat porous to relatively non-permeable (Bertalanffy, 1973; Senge, 2006).

Systems can have any number of defining characteristics. They can be large or small, fragile or robust, relatively stable or highly changeable, tightly or loosely coupled, tractable or intractable, effective or ineffective, and innovative or conservative. Systems are dynamic and can function over a variety of time frames; at any one point they may be in a stage of growth, maintenance or decline.

Systems can be multilevel, with sub-systems differing in their structural characteristics. They can vary from being hierarchical –

like a predator food chain (Pahl-Wostl, 1997), Maslow's hierarchy of human needs (Maslow, 1943), or the rank order within the military (Lider, 1983) – to exhibiting heterarchical properties, whereby they are horizontally overlapping or nested within the larger system of which they form a part. They can be networked, as in the way kinship clusters in traditional societies, or professional collegiality does in modern organisations. Organisations (see Lorenz, 2001, for instance) have horizontal cliques, factions and other informal groupings within and alongside formal departments. In large organisations the departments can be embedded in more extended networks heterarchically, which are in turn part of a hierarchical structure. An organisation may in turn be a component of a large multinational company, which itself is one organisation inside an industry.

These types of multi-scaled, diverse, networked, interactive, hierarchical and heterarchical systems are often termed 'complex'. In a complex system behaviour cannot easily be predicted, and perturbations in one locale may propagate through the levels, or laterally, manifesting as outcomes in an area unrelated in time or place to the originating activity.

Complex systems exhibit properties of emergence – spontaneous behaviours generated from relatively simple interactions – and adaptation over time. When we speak of a CAS, we mean one that is multifaceted, displaying intrinsic laws or principles such as self-organisation, emergent behaviour and capacity to learn or evolve temporally (Ellis and Herbert, 2011; Zhao et al., 2011).

Collectivities as different as biological species, ant colonies, stock markets, the environment, human brains and industrial organisations are CASs, and share similar characteristics. They consist of multiple agents or nodes, at differing levels, resulting in a multiplicity of interactions over space and time.

The agents in human CASs are thought of as 'intelligent'; that is, capable of responding and evolving, which we know as 'adaptive capacity' (Smit and Wandel, 2006). They tend to self-organise, bottom-up. The complexity of the relationships, and the independence and interdependence of the agents' actions, often means that behaviour is hard to predict. Their current behaviours are affected by historical events. Systems and sub-systems can – and do – longitudinally react and adapt to changing circumstances. Iterating behaviours of agents create feedback loops, often delayed, that stimulate further knowledge and change. Agents in specific localities are unable to apprehend all behaviours of those in other parts of large systems, or the system as a whole.

Health Care as a CAS Phenomenon

Health care is a powerful exemplar of the CAS phenomenon. It is an open, large, and broadly effective system characterised by herding, emergent behaviour and adaptation over time. Different parts can be fragile or robust, stable or changeable, differentially coupled, or relatively risky or risk-averse, and these features can vary by time, setting or sub-system.

Modern health care systems are composed of many interacting and interwoven professionals, patients, managers and policy makers, artefacts, equipment and technologies. They consume large amounts of society's resources and are multilayered, heterarchically nested, and ever-changing, producing multiple kinds of outputs and outcomes we variously call 'care', 'treatment', 'interventions' and 'procedures'. Unintended outcomes (Wilson et al., 1999) may also emerge, such as health care-associated harm (Kohn, Corrigan and Donaldson, 2000).

Health services span multiple sub-sectors including aged care, mental health care, acute care, rehabilitation, alternative medicine and community care. Delivery of services takes place in identifiable settings such as aged care facilities, hospitals, health centres, clinics and private practices. Participants cluster; they herd, paying heed to what others are doing. They emulate others, and congregate in groups labelled, for example, the operating room, the paediatric ward and the medical profession. A wide range of caring or support roles are performed by different kinds of medical, nursing and allied health staff, and ancillary and support personnel. In developed countries the costs hover at around 10 per cent of gross domestic product (OECD, 2011); in the USA – an outlier – this has risen to 17 per cent (Bradley et al., 2011).

Many researchers examine health care using linear paradigms and methodologies such as before and after studies or randomised controlled trials (RCTs). These can be critiqued from a CAS vantage point for being reductionist, focused on counting rather than understanding things, failing to recognise interconnections, and attempting to hold variables constant when such a feat is not feasible in ever dynamic health care settings. Complexity theorists, implementation scientists, translational researchers, social scientists and Safety-II experts tend to decry such linear conceptualisations, favouring complex adaptive descriptions and network approaches to examining health care systems. They believe that the whole is not only greater than the parts, but qualitatively different from the sum of the components. So breaking down CASs to understand them will provide an incomplete picture at best, and will mask interactive complexity. No satisfactory account of health care can ignore network effects or systems interconnectivity.

Illuminating Key CAS Characteristics of Health Care

Entire books could be written on the topic 'Health care as a complex adaptive system', but we have chosen three distinctive facets of health care to deepen our understanding of them through a CAS lens. These are: self-organisation (which we contrast with top-down organisational principles); emergent behaviour (specifically looking at overlapping and nested cultures and subcultures); and gaps in the health care CAS (particularly as barriers to integrated, joined-up care). To provide context and sharpen our focus, we present three case studies from our empirical work, each highlighting a hierarchical layer: the agent level, analysing health professionals' behaviours within a mental health service; the departmental level, in a case drawing on research in an emergency department (ED); and the organisational systems level, synthesised from a large-scale research project across an entire health system.

Case 1: Mental Health Professionals' Microsystem Conceptualisations of Patient Safety (Agent Level)

A six-month mixed-method study of two teams within an Australian metropolitan mental health service was undertaken during 2011. The study explored professional conceptualisations and practical accomplishments of patient safety in this setting (Plumb et al., 2011). Structured and unstructured observations of the everyday work of one community service and one acute psychiatric inpatient unit were conducted, as well as in-depth interviews, and a social network analysis and survey of 58 staff members.

A key influence on the framing of this work was Latour's (2005) notion that social institutions are the unstable products of ever-evolving and fragile 'assemblages' of effortful interaction between agents, which can be human and non-human. We found the operation of such emergent assemblages to be the principal mechanism producing patient safety in these settings.

Analysis of the talk and work of the mental health professionals revealed that considerable and repeated effort is made to maintain the functioning of what Mesman (2009) called a 'safety net'. In this setting, the safety net is a dynamic, evolving system of people and things that collectively accomplish the monitoring and intervention work required to keep patients safe. This informal safety system operates in an uncertain environment, in which the impact of any intervention on the safety of a patient is contextually and individually dependent, and where risk is highly unpredictable. The achievement of safe care is always fragile and so considerable redundancy is built in to improve the strength and resilience of the safety net. The professionals cannot know about the whole system in which they work, but can usually do a good enough job to keep their part of the system safe using their bounded, local rationality (Simon, 1955; Simon, 1979; Dekker, 2011a). This research illustrates the importance of an improvised, responsive approach to the task of producing safe care in a context of unpredictability, as well as the constant, moment-by-moment effort required of professionals to maintain it.

Case 2: The Emergency Department as an Interacting CAS Component (Department Level)

An ethnographic study was executed, involving more than a year of observations in the EDs of two tertiary referral hospitals in Sydney, Australia, between 2005 and 2007. The findings showed that emergency clinicians are responsible for guiding the patient's trajectories of care through various overlapping stages that are simultaneously clinical and organisational (Nugus and Braithwaite, 2010). These are: triaging on the basis of urgency of condition; assessment; diagnosis; commencement or completion of the treatment plan; and disposition, usually in the form of in-patient admission or discharge. Most literature regards this journey in a linear fashion – as a 'continuity of care' problem.

The findings noted, however, that the interactions with staff from different occupations, departments and organisations were crucial to making decisions throughout these phases. Care was not delivered merely in the ED, but as a negotiation of the relationships between emergent individual elements, sub-systems across formal occupational and organisational boundaries, and broader level system influences from the patient's initial arrival at the ED.

Observations of 24 medical ward rounds showed that answering three key questions implicitly captures and defines patient pathways in the ED. First, can this patient be discharged or do they need to be admitted as an in-patient to the hospital? Second, if they need admission, where and under whose management should they be transferred, and when? Third, if they can be discharged, how can this be done safely and efficiently (Nugus et al., 2010)? Various interconnected agents, in conglomerations of varying boundary strength, are key reference points in decisions throughout the patient journey in the ED. Understanding the ED as a CAS draws attention to the point that ED care is about managing, through communication, the constantly shifting boundaries between the ED and other agents, sub-systems and systems (Nugus et al., 2010); and the patient journey is not well described as 'linear'.

Case 3: A Socio-ecological Perspective on Emergent Inter-professional Practices across Health Care (Systems Level)

Over a four-year period (2007–2010), we deployed a social science research team to a health system to conduct action research, aiming to stimulate greater levels of inter-professional collaboration (Braithwaite et al., 2013). The health system in the Australian Capital Territory comprised almost 5,000 staff serving a geographic population of around 352,000 people, and provided acute, aged care, rehabilitation, mental health, cancer and community-based services.

The research design was based on socio-ecological theory, aiming to induce improvements to inter-professionalism through multiple interventions. In conjunction with participating staff, the research team conducted 101 substantial improvement activities with 573 participants, 108 feedback sessions with 1,010 participants, 25 educational workshops with 594 participants and 38 other interventional activities with 230 participants. Inevitably, many were conducted in organisational silos, separated from each other.

Despite this longitudinal activity, and the logging of many successful examples of enhanced inter-professional collaboration, attitudes to the quality of inter-professional care, doctor centrality, teamwork and professional identity did not change markedly over the second, third and fourth years of the project. This study showed how hard it is to change health professional attitudes and entrenched ways of working through external means, although it is relatively easy to run separate projects and education sessions. Systems change is enormously challenging for all sorts of reasons, including pre-existing ways of working, resistance to change, and extant professional differences. Health care CASs operate often within contexts that are relatively unknowable and difficult to influence, notwithstanding efforts to change them: they self-organise, exhibit spontaneous behaviours, and adapt over time, regardless of initiatives specifically designed to alter them.

All in all, the cases highlighted CAS characteristics including self-organisation, heterarchy, hierarchy, adaptation and adaptive capacity, herding and networking. Particularly in Case 1, we observed emergent behaviours reflected in everyday, spontaneous interactive practices. In Case 2, we saw complexity and dynamism as compared with simplistic linearity across adjacent interacting cultures. Gaps and silos, and resistance to external change, were notable in Case 3.

Next, to tease out some of these, we put self-organisation, emergence and culture, and gaps in the health care CAS under the microscope.

The Health Care CAS under a Microscope

Self-organisation

With self-organisation (Mennin, 2010), coordinated activities and structural characteristics emerge, and forms of order become manifest, without any single source of central or top-down control, to meet system goals. This is a feature of health care, because clinicians are generally well-trained professionals with considerable autonomy and discretion, and they make relatively independent decisions in providing care to individual patients, typically within loosely coordinated networks.

Many of the behavioural repertoires and professionalised structures arise from the way clinicians organise themselves into groups, most of which is based on specialisation. Thus everywhere we observe groups of specialised physicians, surgeons and pathologists (to mention only three) collectively organising themselves and offering services via public or private business models, depending on the country and circumstances. We also observe informal local clinical networks spontaneously emerging, such as those reflecting friendships, trust, support mechanisms, referral patterns and working conveniences. Cases 1 and 2 remind us of this. A crucial feature of the sum of the interactions is that things for the most part are kept safe. Millions of decisions are made, tasks performed, treatments administered, procedures conducted, tests reviewed, work processed, care provided and patients treated, without mishap.

Clinicians are collectively organised at the systems level, too, and can network together to resist external pressures, as in Case 3. They can also lobby or influence others, exercising power and influence in their relationships with politicians, providers, policy-makers, regulators and others. They do this through vehicles – including colleges and associations – that represent their views and interests.

However, health care is also subject to public interest considerations, and other stakeholders are involved. The public, governments, payers, and health insurers have an interest, and want to have a say, in the system. Their 'say' often takes the form of top-down regulatory demands, which stand in stark contrast to bottom-up, localised organisational behaviours. This phenomenon is not peculiar to health care. The top-down, central 'command-and-control' tendencies of those in authority meeting the bottom-up, 'leave-me-alone-to-get-on-with-the-real-work' proclivities of independently-minded 'coalface' workers in systems is well known. It manifests particularly in other professionalised environments such as accounting practices, academic departments, consulting companies and legal partnerships.

Modern health systems have in recent decades received attention from regulators, policy-makers, insurers and accreditors because of greater recognition of iatrogenesis, the desire to improve quality of care and patient safety, and the requirements of many authorities for greater accountability and efficiency. Regulation takes multiple forms, but broadly involves constraining or enabling various behaviours, and assigning responsibilities and accountabilities to people providing care. In health care it typically involves promulgating laws, policies, standards, goals, targets and indicators to shape system and sub-system behaviours. Regulation can be mandatory or voluntary, and often takes the form of co-regulation, where multiple parties have a role to play in exercising authority, assigning accountability, specifying requirements and delivering systems outcomes.

Cook and Woods (1994) point out that the top-down authorities, agencies and bureaucracies function at the blunt end of the system; they do not directly keep things safe, but they do act when errors are made. By contrast, those at the sharp end, providing direct care, for the most part keep things safe moment to moment, day by day. When things go wrong, they get swept up and often blamed by a review or enquiry (Hughes, Travaglia and Braithwaite, 2010; Hindle et al., 2006) sponsored or run by those at the blunt end, particularly if, with hindsight bias, the 'errors' are seen as 'preventable'. All in all, self-organisation contributes to CAS resilience by providing a bonded cohort of interacting agents, departmental interactions and systems-wide efforts contributing everyday tasks to the safety profile of patient care. Case 1 supports these contentions, and reflects the enactment of safety.

Emergence and Culture

As agents within systems interact, jostle with, and influence each other, participating in all sorts of political and cultural exchanges, they exhibit and produce emergent behaviours. Agents (clinical staff, ancillary and support staff, and managers) actively participate in what Strauss et al. (1963) and Strauss (1978) called 'the negotiated order' – a term coined to emphasise the way that people parley, confer and make trade-offs in meeting their individual and group objectives. These politically and culturally informed exchanges go a long way towards describing the organisational dynamics underpinning the processes of providing care. Case 2 neatly brings this out in emergency care and the cross-boundary intentions of the ED and other units.

What we mean by culture is the collective attitudes, values, behaviours and practices of a given human cluster (Braithwaite, 2005). It is a kind of unseen glue that binds people – unseen, that is, by the people in the culture who have accommodated to it, or been socialised in it, and to whom it is a taken for granted, 'normal' way of being and doing. Behaviours tend to stabilise to a recognisable degree, showing distinctive patterning. Cultures can be nurturing, productive, helpful and supportive – but also they can be toxic, politically charged, prejudiced and disabling, or an incredibly dense mixture of these and other features (Braithwaite, 2005; Braithwaite, Hyde and Pope, 2010).

Boundaries circumscribing health care cultures are typically porous, denoting a degree of interdependence between agents interacting within the environment of any CAS. Much social research has shown that agents within cultures and across sub-cultures are mutually influencing (Barnes, 2001; Nugus, 2008) – affecting each other, and shaping and attenuating behaviours, sometimes quite extensively (Braithwaite, 2006). Thus, in Case 2, ED clinicians inter-related with each other and also tried to influence staff in other units to take patients. Out of these interactive behaviours and iterative influences arise cultural and sub-cultural features, which take the shape of unique, localised patterns in the organisational landscape. These manifest as multiple informal behavioural repertoires e.g., friendships, in-groups, alliances, coalitions, *ad hoc* teams and informal groups

(Eljiz, Fitzgerald and Sloan, 2010; McMahon, MacCurtain and O'Sullivan, 2010).

Sub-cultures, then, interact within and seek to affect each other. Those working in a health care organisation notice this. Over time, sub-cultures act and react in response to altered circumstances *vis à vis* other sub-cultures. Yet paradoxically it does not seem that organisational life is unstable or unfathomable: organisations for the most part are not excessively unruly or out of control, and, to a considerable degree, the sub-cultures exhibit levels of stability – not just at particular points in time (Allen, 2000), but longitudinally. This is the difference between organised and disorganised complexity, and how we can have organisations and their constituent units at all. Otherwise, they would be constantly disorganised – even dissolving, reappearing and reforming in a dizzying, ambiguous and perplexing mixture, like folding and refolding pizza dough. They may be like this some of the time, but cultures are also decidedly consistent for the most part.

Culture and sub-cultures are not only heterarchically overlapping, but nested (for an example, see the box below). Martin (2002) has mobilised three perspectives on culture which can be deployed to tease out its nested nature. There can be the overarching cultural features of the whole organisation such as a teaching hospital, or aged care facility, which at this macro-level can exhibit dominant features such as being productive, collaborative, corrupt or toxic, for example. There can at the intermediate, meso-level be groupings such as wards, units or departments or less formal microsystems, groupings of friends, or referral networks, each with distinctive features in broad alignment with or at cross purposes to the larger prevailing culture. And there can be even more localised cultural features expressed by small-scale cliques, elite groupings, work friends, closed circles, those with enmities or hostilities, lunch crowds or in-groups and out-groups.

Highlighting Nested Behaviours

People inside organisations are simultaneously members of multiple groupings. An individual can be a woman, a doctor, a paediatrician, and a friend of others making up one of her in-groups; a mentor to paediatricians-in-training, a subordinate to the head of department, and someone with an identifiable group of specialist colleagues to whom her patients are referred when necessary. She can be working across wards 1a and 6b, and spend time in outpatient clinics and neonatal intensive care when necessary, in a hospital which is simultaneously part of a university-health science alliance, a regional grouping, and a chain of providers. She can also run a free clinic in a deprived area once a week, and be a member of a high-powered paediatric college committee and a scientific advisory body planning an annual research conference with senior colleagues.

She is simultaneously not, amongst other things, a member of various cultural groups including men or the nursing profession, and she is not part of the anaesthetics department, the senior management team, or many other departments, services and in-groups. Her swirl of sub-cultural memberships and non-memberships is considerable, even bewildering. She transitions across multiple, nested sub-cultures in the space of even a few hours in a busy day.

All these emergent behaviours make health care difficult to fathom, devilishly hard to manage, challenging for staff to navigate, bewildering for patients to access or understand, and never-endingly interesting for their inhabitants, and researchers and commentators on them. It also means that health care CASs and their constituent components are overlapping and nested, with sub-cultures inside of, and juxtaposed with reference to, other sub-structures and sub-cultures. The metaphor of a Russian doll comes to mind when thinking about the nested nature of these features of health care CASs, and multiple interrelating Russian dolls when thinking of the overlapping interactions of sub-cultures.

Gaps in the Health Care CAS

Cases 2 and 3 particularly show examples of gaps – between organisational units, as in Case 2, and that projects are frequently managed in silos, as in Case 3. Opportunities to understand systems arise from examining circumstances in which they fail to be joined up or integrated, looking at what happens in the system's cracks. A recent systematic review (Braithwaite, 2010) of literature on social spaces, divides and holes (collectively, gaps) in health care found only 13 studies, showing how under-represented the study of gaps is. This review noted the prevalence of the gap phenomenon. The spaces, holes and disjunctions between departments, wards and units, between organisations offering care services and between professional tribes are not just common, but largely define the social and professional structures that people inhabit in health care.

Most people work comfortably within their groups or localised organisational structures, and many do not have the inclination or time to reach out across organisational, professional, cultural or departmental divides. Often, agents in one part of a system, for structural, geographical, financial, functional or political reasons, are not aware of the work of others. In some cases, ties between silos have been severed; in others relationships are weak; in yet others there is occasional interaction; and in still others there is close involvement of two or more groups or entities (Cook, Render and Woods, 2000). It may be the case that decentralisation of health care structures in many systems, driven by technology, innovation and pervasive restructuring (Braithwaite, Runciman and Merry, 2009), has exacerbated the gaps in health care. However, a key point is that in all health systems there are limits to connectivity, and in the real world the behaviours of participants can be frayed, antagonistic, or dissolve at the edges of their social and professional groupings.

An example of naturally occurring gaps lies with the tribalism of clinical professionals (Braithwaite, 2005). Clinicians tend to relate to their professional reference group (doctors with doctors, nurses with nurses, allied health staff with allied health staff) rather than form multidisciplinary teams (Braithwaite and Westbrook, 2005; Braithwaite et al. [in press]). Homophily seems to be widespread. Creating joined-up, integrated health care, across organisational and professional divides, appears to be at odds with the way health systems work in practice, particularly on wards and in hospitals (Milne, 2012). This may be different in sectors such as mental health (Plumb, 2012) and rehabilitation (Pereira, 2013) settings, where there may be higher degrees of multi-disciplinarity, team orientation, and fewer groups and divides. But overall, there are manifold gaps in health care, and they manifest as threats to system resilience. Palpably, people, patients, information and trust can fall through the cracks in – or fail to bridge gaps across – the health system, introducing unspecified risks to effective care. In the cases we presented, gaps, boundaries and discontinuities were seen amongst the dynamic behaviours manifesting as networks and cultures.

Discussion

What are the Improvement Strategies to Which the CAS View Leads?

Health care, then, exemplifies the properties of CASs and how they behave. We can see many characteristics of CASs in our analysis of health care, and our case studies depicting their features at agent, departmental and organisational-wide levels. A particularly hard game, harder than chess or even decoding the genome, is how to 'improve' health systems. Health care CASs are highly complicated and self-determining. It is extremely difficult to describe them satisfactorily, let alone influence them, and even when this is possible, unintended consequences can result. Another hard game is to understand how and where they are resilient, how and why they are safe most of the time, and how – or even whether – we can strengthen that resilience.

In regard to the first game, the short answer is that managers and policy-makers have pressed particularly in recent times to improve health care systems. Efforts have been and are being made to enhance efficiency, the quality of care, and safety for patients. Reformers and improvement agents and agencies have introduced incident management systems (Travaglia, Westbrook and Braithwaite, 2009), safety training programs (Braithwaite et al., 2007), root cause analyses (Iedema et al., 2006) and checklists (Haynes et al., 2011), as well as many projects such as hand washing, handovers and improvement teams (Braithwaite and Coiera, 2010). Newer initiatives have been encouraged by the demonstration of occasional successes, and much ingenuity has been spent striving to learn from these, attempting to diffuse ideas, models and strategies, and hoping that across time people can provide resources, support and facilitation to make further improvements. Even so, there will always be adverse consequences from improvement activities to CASs, and past experience suggests uptake of any enhancements will be patchy. And even patchy gains take time. Indeed, while there have been celebrated initiatives such as using checklists in theatres (Haynes et al., 2011), creating medical emergency teams (METs) to address deterioration of a patient's condition (Hillman et al., 2005) and reducing central line infections in intensive care units (Pronovost et al., 2006a), there is no known study demonstrating across-the-board, step-change improvements in health care safety and quality. That these notable initiatives are celebrated demonstrates the point, and there is an increasing view that the level of improvement across systems has been disappointing considering the effort put in (e.g. Wachter, 2010).

As to our second game, resilience to system perturbations is characterised by a high degree of adaptive capacity – where adaptive capacity is the ability of systems, sub-systems and agents to learn and respond to changing environments or work pressures, and bounce back from problems. Adaptive capacity is particularly critical in environments such as health care, which display high variability. The unpredictability of a disturbance – in timing, magnitude, duration and character – means that clinicians must be continually aware, flexible and ready to act. Yet most are busy providing care, and are not routinely or concertedly working – at least not 'formally' – on projects explicitly targeted at improving the system. They are maintaining the system safely, for the most part, as in Case 1, but not always, or specifically, 'improving it' by running projects or initiatives dreamed up by the top-down authorities, as in Case 3.

We can see adaptive behaviours in the activities of the individual agents in Case 1 in the mental health service (Plumb et al., 2011), where an informally developed pattern of monitoring, intervention and redundancy emerges to create a safer environment. This is typical of many parts of health systems. Noone sanctioned this, or insisted on it; like the Nike advertisement, clinicians 'just do it'. Similar adaptive behaviours by individuals in emergency departments manifest as they interact with other inpatient services to create strategies to meet the requirements of patient care (Nugus and Braithwaite, 2010) in a resource-limited environment. The system-wide case, number 3, (Braithwaite et al. [in press]; see also Runciman et al.,

2012b) draws out yet another aspect pertinent to improvement: external agents cannot necessarily induce greater enhancements to systems. In reality, it takes a village.

How Can the Resilience Characteristics of Health Care be Improved by Seeing Health Care as a CAS?

Resilience, even if it is not given this name, is a natural property of health care CASs (e.g. Braithwaite, Runciman and Merry, 2009). In the Case 1, agent-level study, and at the point where levels of care come together departmentally in Case 2, there appear to be elements of resilience. This seems to be what clinicians, if left to their own devices, do: create a system where most things go right, sometimes in tandem with, and sometimes despite, the formalised improvement initiatives, projects and systems sanctioned from above.

By way of contrast, the organisation-wide context of Case 3 highlights widespread resistance. We discussed earlier the importance of defining the system perimeter. If we define the boundary as the hospital, for example, the resistance to change might be viewed in relation to an *externally imposed* change initiative. Thus, even though the Case 3 project was a lateral collaboration of researchers and clinicians with managerial approval for the research partnership, it may still be framed by shopfloor clinical participants as invasive and not under their direction. Here, clinicians' attitudes in Case 3 did not alter over time, despite longitudinal efforts to enhance levels of inter-professionalism.

As predicted by the CAS characteristics we have laid out here, the health care system is constantly changing internally, as new behaviours emerge to satisfy the requirements of day-to-day patient care. For example, clinicians frequently create workarounds to deal with unforeseen situations, time pressures or scarce resources. So, in reality, if a change initiative is viewed as an external perturbation, and imposed on the internal culture by a foreign culture, then the system can be quite resilient in its ability to resist the threatening forces of the change (for better or worse).

In each of these case studies we can also observe the self-organisation principles at work, sometimes complementing and sometimes counterbalancing the top-down tendencies. The micro-behaviours in the mental health setting show how safety is enacted by the staff themselves, often through an entirely separate and additional set of activities to that mandated by those in authority. We can see the resilience properties of CASs emerging in these examples. The multiple and unique paths created to solve each individual problem also create multiple and unique opportunities for failure. And we can see how the multiple methods and overlapping strategies used to deal with the challenges outlined in each case have, often inadvertently, added system complexity.

Cultures, and sub-cultures, too, pose interesting challenges for health care resilience. If culture is something an organisation or system has (Smircich, 1983) – a variable like other variables such as the organisational structure, the human resources policies or the IT capability – then in principle it is able to be manipulated, shaped or influenced. In the process of doing this, it may be that resilience can be sharpened or enhanced by managers, regulators, insurers, or government. But if culture is something an organisation or system *is* – a fundamental, defining core of that organisation or system – then it is not readily changed by agents external to the clinical coalface, even through the concerted efforts of multiple stakeholders. Our cases suggest the latter: culture is something that defines an organisation or system, something it *is* rather than something it *has*. On the basis of parallel logic, resilience might also be a core attribute of an organisation rather than a variable subject to manipulation. If this is so, then the cultural, sub-cultural and resilience settings of any health care organisation cannot readily be changed by external stakeholders' requirements, policymakers' pronouncements or managerialist actions. Self-organisation and adaptive capacity then become the crucial determinant of on-going success.

PART II
The Locus of Resilience – Individuals, Groups, Systems

Chapter 7
Resilience in Intensive Care Units: The HUG Case

Jean Pariès, Nicolas Lot, Fanny Rome and Didier Tassaux

Introduction

The intensive care unit (ICU) of the University Hospital of Geneva (HUG) is a big unit which resulted from the merger in 2005 of two hitherto separate services. This merger triggered an organisational crisis that developed over a few years. Despite this, the actual performance of the unit improved in terms of care quantity, quality, and patient safety. In other words, the unit proved to be resilient. At the request of the unit we undertook, in 2010, a qualitative study to understand better the reasons for this resilience. The expectation was that this would allow the unit to consolidate and improve its strategies. We used an interpretative framework based on the concept of resilience engineering to observe how the ICU was functioning, and we tried to understand how and why it seemed to succeed (or fail) in controlling variations, disturbances and destabilisation during this period. We also aimed at discussing and complementing that conceptual framework through the ICU experience.

Background: The ICU Context

Intensive care units (ICUs) are complex adaptive systems (Cook, 1998), a land of the unexpected and uncertainties. They manage high-risk patients, for whom one or several of their vital functions usually necessitate pharmacological and technical support. Services are 'intensive' because they require significant resources in terms of workforce (e.g., one nurse for two patients) and highly sophisticated equipment (e.g., monitoring tools, artificial breathing apparatus). Due to the high costs involved, resources do not account for operational workload peaks and the complexity of extreme clinical conditions (Tassaux et al., 2008). Consequently, staff frequently face overload episodes that exceed the unit's operational capacity. Care processes are also subjected to numerous unpredictable events due to the random occurrence of various pathologies, significant uncertainties regarding the evolution of patients' conditions, and limitations of medical knowledge in the face of the complexity of some pathologies. Hence, many of the care processes are under-specified and staff are regularly pushing their boundaries. Adding to the difficulty, the lack of care production may be more dangerous than the lack of care precaution. Last, but not least, the work environment creates many economic, political, and psychological pressures, because of the high unit cost of the care processes, the sensitivity of the population to this kind of advanced medicine, its media exposure, the interface of ICU with other inpatient units, and because of the constant interaction with patients' families.

The ICU system (including individuals, work groups and the service as a whole) therefore has no other choice than to adapt (Anders et al., 2006). Several mechanisms are triggered in order to maintain an even performance level (in terms of care provision, quality and safety) despite the regular and possibly severe deteriorations of operational conditions (Cook, 1998). The balance between predefined responses and creative ones in particular appears to be one of the key features of these strategies. But many questions remain about the underlying mechanisms that allow that balance to maintain the performance–risk ratio within a range acceptable for shareholders and society, despite all the disturbances.

A Surprising Performance

The HUG-ICU has features of particular interest for those studying these mechanisms. With 36 beds and about 350 staff, it is a large ICU. More importantly, it resulted from the merger (in October 2005) of two hitherto separate services: surgical intensive care and internal medicine intensive care. These two services had a history of competition, if not of conflict. The two managers were rivals, and differed greatly in their methods of management, the relationships they encouraged between doctors and nurses, and so on. The head of the former internal medicine ICU was designated as the head of the newly formed service, as the other manager was retiring. The four medical assistants to each of the two former heads of service were combined to form a team of eight deputy heads of the new service, but they initially failed to collaborate and form a cohesive team. The new service struggled to find its legitimacy or direction and a growing uneasiness emerged among staff, especially nurses. The turnover of nurses increased to alarming rates (about 30 per cent per year), and so did absenteeism. Seventeen per cent of caregivers had a significantly higher burnout score two years after the merger.

Despite all these difficulties, the overall performance of the service increased significantly. More patients were admitted, representing a 20 per cent increase in productivity over the first two years. Peak hours were well handled and re-admission rates decreased. The efficiency and the quality of care improved. While the severity of the clinical status of admitted patients (SAP) remained very high (one of the worse average SAPs in Switzerland), the new service reached one of the best outcomes: only 0.75 per cent of the SAPsS predicted deaths.

So, why was the HUG–ICU able to overcome the profound disturbances caused by the merger? A few members of the unit management team began to ask themselves this question, hoping that a better understanding of these success mechanisms would enable the service to stabilise gains, and hopefully to build further improvements, including for day-to-day operations planning and setting, as well as to design planned diagnostics for other ICUs. Consequently, they decided to look into this question with the assistance of external consultants.

The Conceptual Framework

The research project was launched with an explicit reference to the notion of resilience engineering (Hollnagel, Woods and Leveson, 2006), which offered a relevant and innovative conceptual framework to address the issue of managing disturbance.[1] Resilience engineering suggests a different view of the traditional relationship between variation and performance. While classical performance enhancement approaches seek to reduce the frequency and amplitude of (internal or external) variations the system is exposed to, resilience engineering aims at improving the system's ability to handle variations and perturbations. It asserts that classical approaches cannot fully succeed in eradicating variations in a complex system, but tend to dismantle the diversity of available responses, and thus the system's ability to face the unexpected (Pariès, 2011). The resilience engineering concept also encourages a rethinking of the organisation and its processes, the cooperation and competences in order to develop capabilities for managing variations and disturbances.

Hollnagel (2010) proposes a list of four capabilities that enable the understanding of the system's resilience characteristics from a viewpoint relatively close to the robustness of the system's control function to cope with disturbances: (1) the system must respond in an appropriate manner in real time (including when coping with the unexpected); (2) it must have an adequate surveillance capability; (3) it must be forward-looking, anticipating what can happen and preparing responses; (4) it must be able to learn from its experience. Woods (2010) proposes a list of capabilities inspired by adaptability management ideals. Among others, the system's resilience is conditional upon the capabilities of recognising that its adaptation capabilities are collapsing or will become inadequate considering future bottlenecks; recognising the threat of exhausting its buffers or stocks; detecting any necessary change of priority for the management of objectives trade-offs; changing its viewpoint, varying any perspectives that go beyond the nominal states of the system; recognising the need for learning new ways to adapt.

From a more organisational perspective, the high reliability organisations (HRO) community (Rochlin, La Port and Roberts, 1987) tried to define the features that are shared by organisations

1 Resilience can be defined as the system's ability to maintain its integrity and its performance, at least partially, while under internal or external variations and disturbances (i.e. pressures, constraints, failures, errors, violations, hazards), whether nominal, extreme or exceptional.

that seem to be highly reliable in their management of safety. The HRO trend has shown that such organisations do not follow a bureaucratic hierarchical structure but are, rather, characterised by both a powerful centralised and strategic decision making process (i.e. consistent with the classical hierarchical model), and a decentralised operational decision making process, which empowers operators at the bottom, for safety issues in particular. This leads to the polycentric governance idea generalised by Ostrom (2010), which means that the ecosystem governance is ensured by multiple authority centres rather than by a unified one.

One additional important dimension refers to the management of objectives. Organisations usually have multiple and partially contradictory objectives: e.g., a care unit has efficiency, budgets, delay reductions, patient safety, care quality, care accessibility and patient focus objectives. The organisations' attempt to balance their performance to achieve these different objectives in a bounded world makes trade-offs necessary. Resilience somehow measures the quality and robustness of these trade-offs, i.e., their stability in the presence of disturbances. In this respect, an important resilience characteristic is the ability to make sacrificing decisions, such as accepting the failure to reach an objective in the short term to ensure another long term objective, or 'cutting one's losses' by giving up initial ambitions (e.g., planned therapeutic objectives) to save what is essential.

Method

As already stated, we used an interpretative framework of the organisation inspired by resilience engineering to observe the HUG–ICU's functions, and to verify if it would be possible through this lens to understand how and why the ICU seemed to succeed (and on some measures, to fail) to control the variations, disturbances and destabilisations it faced. The research was structured into five steps, as described below.

Step 1: Clarification of the Conceptual Framework

The first step consisted in defining more precisely the organisational resilience concept and clarifying its relevance to the issue to be addressed by the HUG–ICU. We attempted to merge the approaches referred to in the previous section, and complemented them with the psychological and sociological viewpoint at the workplace (Alter, 2007). We also tried to clarify the interactions between different organisational levels (e.g., individuals and teams, teams and departments, base and hierarchy, departments and the overall organisation) from a resilience perspective. As Woods (2006) pointed out, the resilience at a certain organisation level is influenced or even determined by the interactions of this level with others. However, the resilience literature seldom mentions any relationship between resilience at different organisational levels. For example, does the resilience at a higher level imply resilience at lower levels, and vice versa? A synthesis of the literature on stress, burnout and suffering at work suggests that the link between operators' stress and objective work constraints is complex. A significant level of difficulty at work can only be sustained by a notable personal commitment that must correspond to individual values (i.e., feelings of being useful, work quality). These values must map onto those developed by the organisation, and be reinforced during the selection process of its members. In addition, the work group plays an essential role since it can help in reasserting the real purpose of the job as well as its constraints, while facilitating exchanges and communication.

Step 2: A Resilience Observation Framework

The second step focused on transforming these conceptual resilience principles into an interpretative framework that could allow for the detection, amongst the characteristics of the ICU, of the properties that correspond to those described in the theoretical frame of reference. We have developed an observation grid by combining Hollnagel's and Wood's resilience capabilities lists, complemented by the perspectives discussed above. We also attempted to discriminate the resilient characteristics associated with normal, disturbed and crisis situations, while keeping in mind that the boundaries between these states are fuzzy. This led us towards the establishment of a resilience observation framework, shown in extract in Table 7.1.

Table 7.1 Organisational resilience conditions extract

	Predetermination	Coupling to reality	Feedback	
	Management of goals and constraints, modelling and anticipation	*Surveillance, perception, understanding*	*Responsiveness*	*Feedback regarding the system, the adaptations and the learning process*
Normal	*Objectives, values, trade-off principles* *System models* *Risks & disturbances model* *Safety model* *Predefined responses repertoire* *Anticipated 'margins of manoeuvre'* *Trust*	*Monitoring processes* *Attention pattern* *Sentinel events* *Signals of anomaly* *Signals of loss of control* *Stress, fear, anxiety* *Self-monitoring* *Mutual monitoring* *Surveillance of the surveillance efficiency*	*Competences, routines, procedures, skills, know-how* *Efficiency thoroughness trade-off* *Cooperation*	*Organisational lucidity on real activities* A posteriori *update of risk and safety model* *Re-adaptation of rules, protocols, procedures* *Re-engineering of the rule making process*
Disturbance emergency	*Same as above +:* *Alerting signals list* *Model of the loss of control signals* *Anticipation of the alternative/recovery/ backup solutions* *Recovery modes*	*Same as above +:* *Surveillance of the alerting signals* *Warning priority hierarchies* *Surveillance of the loss of control signals* *Surveillance of the recovery signals*	*Same as above +:* *Functional adaptation* *Prioritisation, shift of goals, trade-offs* *Cooperation adaptation* *Creativeness*	*Same as above +:* *Debriefing* *Collective analysis* *Expert analysis* *Evolution/ adaptation of competences, high level values, ethics and meta-rules* *Trust levels update*
Crisis	*Same as above +:* *Emergency modes* *Definition of the vital functions* *Objectives adaptation* *Stocks and buffers management* *Withdrawal/back-up strategies*	*Same as above +:* *Perception of the loss of control*	*Same as above +:* *Change in the viewpoint or strategy* *Stocks, buffers, margins, tolerances* *Restructuring of the work group,* *Sacrificing decisions* *Creativeness, 'DIY'*	*Same as above +:* *Crisis debriefing* *Coaching*

Step 3: 'Observing'Resilience in the ICU

The third step consisted in applying these observation elements to the functioning of ICUs. We developed a translation dictionary to link the resilience engineering lexicon to the ICU's operations lexicon. Then, Table 7.1 was instantiated at three organisational levels:

1. the unit level
2. the team level
3. the individual operator's level

This instantiated table was used to conduct interviews with ICU experts in order to detect phenomena (e.g., processes, activities, behaviours) that seemed to correspond to one or several functions identified as resilience conditions. These links are summarised in Table 7.2.

The next step defined identifiers and data collection methodologies (observations, interviews, questionnaires) appropriate for the characteristics featured in the above table in order to make an initial assessment of the existing resilience capabilities, to understand the processes upon which they rely, and how the organisation owns – knowingly or not – these capabilities and can maintain them.

Table 7.2 Potential resilience supports for ICU

	Predetermination	Coupling to reality	Feedback	
	Management of goals and constraints, modelling, and anticipation	*Monitoring, perception, understanding*	*Reactivity, responsiveness*	*Feedback regarding the system, adaptation, learning process*
Operators	*Activity of the doctor on duty (DOD)* *Activity of the MAN*[2] *Literature review* *Care quality principles, protocols and good practices*	*Generic monitoring of patient's appearance and behaviour* *Monitoring of displays* *Reference to threshold values*	*Operator competences* *Ability to take initiatives* *Task prioritisation Management of clinical misunderstanding* *Workload management* *Withdrawal rationale*	*Experience building*
Teams	*Medical visit* *Relationship between MAN and DOD* *Pre-visit* *Doctors' symposium*	*Medical visit* *Informal communication* *Solidarity, attention and mutual aid (among peers with the same job or between different jobs)*	*Physicians'–nurses' relationship* *Cooperation between nurses* *Pre-visit, medical visit* *Protocols* *Informal adjustments*	*Teaching of residents by supervisors* *Transfer of competences during medical visits*
Service	*Daily physicians' meeting (anticipation of potential patients' discharge (= 'jokers*[3]*')* *Nurses' assignment* *Pre-visit* *Clearance from duty of some caregivers for reserve resources*	*Duplication of monitoring displays inside the physicians' meeting room* *Visits of cubicles by the MAN*	*Dynamic assignment* *Pre-visit* *Allocation of experienced staff to difficult cases* *Temporary opening of beds within other departments* *Discharge of patients*	*Psychologist* *Team resource management training ('CHLOE'*[4]*)* *User-oriented procedures*

2 The managing assistant nurse (MAN) is a senior nurse dedicated to matching between patients' needs and nurses' resources. Its role consists in monitoring the number of patients' entries and exits and allocating them to staff.

3 Called 'bumpable' patients in Cook (1998).

4 CHLOE is a team resource management program and stands in French for 'Communication, Harmonisation, Leadership, Organisation, Equipe'.

Step 4: Collecting Data

Table 7.3 below summarises the methods that were used, and the resources involved, to carry out the collection of data corresponding to the identifiers noted in the previous step.

Table 7.3 Data collection methods

Target	Data collection method	Issue
MAN	*Work analysis* *Observation of daily walk* *Interviews* *Interviews of colleagues about the MAN's role*	*Nurses' workload anticipation process* *Permanent adjustment process between available nursing resources and the need for nursing resources generated by the patients*
Doctor 'on call'	*Observation and interview*	*Workload management* *Responses to unexpected situations* *Responses to emergency situations*
Medical visit	*Observation*	*Therapeutic project construction and update* *Monitoring of care processes* *Learning and teaching processes* *Real time work flow management* *Mid-term and long term workload anticipation processes*
Doctors' symposium	*Observation*	*Therapeutic project construction and update* *Real-time work flow management* *Mid-term and long term workload anticipation processes*
Medical transmission	*Observation of shift handover*	
Physicians during night shifts	*Observation and interview*	
Resuscitation call process	*Observation*	*Responses to emergency situations*
All staff	*Interviews of a representative sample of the main jobs* *Half-day focus groups with multi-job attendance*	*Workload management* *List of disturbances, threats and destabilising situations* *Response modes to these threats* *Responses to emergency situations*
Nurse in charge of two simultaneous serious patients	*Observation and interview*	*Workload management* *Responses to unexpected situations*
Adverse events reporting and investigation	*Review of documents* *Interviews of people in charge of adverse event analysis*	
System design	*Review of a series of organisation and process design documents*	*Organisational features* *Organisational resilience features*
Performance indicators	*Review and analysis of the relevant performance, quality and safety indicators*	*Level of performance* *Demonstrated resilience capacities*

In practice, we spent 20 days within the service and among the staff at work. Two sub-processes symptomatic of intensive care activity were selected for deeper analysis.

1. the patient flow management
2. the construction and update of the therapeutic project

Step 5: Reaching Conclusions

The fifth and last step aimed at inferring how to improve the assessment and the management of resilience in the ICU. The team of researchers – comprising both internal staff and external consultants – wrote a final report presenting the context, the conceptual framework, the methodology and the findings of the study, which are summarised in the next section of this paper. Presentations to the staff were made within the ICU, within the hospital, and at various conferences in Europe.

Beyond the presentation of the findings, the awareness gained through the research led to the launch by the ICU of a follow-up project called REACT, which was intended to design a specific training aimed at improving the crisis management abilities of the staff.

Findings and Discussion

Anticipation and Work Flow Management

The main regulation tool to address the permanent challenge of adapting the fixed capacity to fluctuating demand relies on the flexibility of the patients' exit rate. Since it is not possible to agree and organise an exit in a timeframe short enough to respond to an entry demand, the process necessarily includes a strong ability to anticipate.

The MAN's role demonstrates this anticipation capacity well. Although the final decision to admit or discharge patients relies on doctors, the MAN's role consists in monitoring, planning and catalysing entries into and exits from the unit. The MAN's actions include attendance at doctors' symposiums to identify patients who can be discharged by the end of the day if need be (called 'jokers'), regular communication with doctors to update such information, visiting cubicles to follow up the care progress and assess the fatigue and stress level of nurses, exchanges with peers from other units within the hospital, constant monitoring of the hospital emergency department's admission planning and of the operating room's planning to identify elective patients (i.e., patients with a reserved post-operation bed at the ICU) and stand-by patients (i.e. patients who require a bed at the ICU but who can wait for one to be vacated). The medical visit is a second key element in the anticipation and constant control of the entry and exit flows. It specifies and gathers the necessary information along various timeframes. Finally, the doctors' symposiums (mornings and evenings) enable the synthesis of this information, the collective elaboration of the required trade-offs (in particular between the admitted or exiting patients' interests).

When this anticipatory regulation process cannot accommodate the demands for care, workload surges and situations of critical peak workload occur. The operating mode then deviates from the system's nominal mode into a kind of crisis mode or emergency mode. These are relatively common situations, requiring the speeding up of the medical visit, requests for additional resources, transfers of patients to the recovery room, delaying entry by keeping patients in the intermediate care unit or in the recovery room, monitoring patients who are transferred 'upstairs', i.e. in their initial unit (e.g., surgery), speeding up exits or delaying them (e.g., by putting patients back to sleep).

A capacity crisis can also occur due to simultaneous critical cases, or temporarily understaffed teams (especially during night shifts). The response basically starts with an over-mobilisation at the bottom of the pyramid upon the call to rescue colleagues' resources, through an over-delegation towards junior staff (e.g., senior physicians towards residents, nurses towards trainee nurses, etc.), a significant mutual aid, and the support of accelerated, shortened or dedicated protocols. A key success factor of such crisis management appears to be the ability to adapt dynamically the level of delegation and decentralisation on the operation floor. Obviously, the management of these adaptations relies heavily on strong requirements for skills and the accuracy of their perception by the team. In other words, competency is a 'constraint that de-constrains' (Alderson and Doyle, 2010). The question of trust plays a central role. Whatever the sophistication of the competence management process, it cannot guarantee the homogeneity of skills in spite of the diversity of curricula and the turnover. It is essential that everyone knows accurately what can and cannot be expected of their colleagues. It is also essential that everyone understands the underlying conditions of a received delegation, in terms of expected expertise, bottom lines, and the ability to recognise that one's limitations have been reached. We could observe numerous and various, subtle and implicit, mechanisms regarding the manifestation and adjustment of this mutual trust. For example, a resident can infer the level of trust the work group shows in him or her from the tasks he or she has been attributed. We could also observe a series of protection envelope 'tricks', such as sentinel events, alerting signals, call-back rules and deviation thresholds that allow those who delegate to keep control of their delegation.

In this kind of situation, trade-offs are necessarily made, especially between the interests of incoming patients and the interests of patients who are kept within the unit but see their care process reduced to release resources, not to mention the 'jokers'. Such trade-offs often represent sacrificing decisions, in the sense that they lead to a global redistribution of care and risk, to the detriment of some patients and to the benefit of others. And this can only be justified by reaching a higher level in the goals–means abstraction hierarchy (e.g., referring to ethical values like justice rather than to a therapeutic protocol or available medical knowledge).

The Medical Visit and the Management of the Clinical Complexity

The medical visit is a central component of the collective development of the therapeutic project. It specifies the objectives with different timeframes; it provides guidance to reach those objectives, clarifies the alerting signals and expected threshold values for clinical parameters or behaviours, while allowing operators to take initiatives when necessary, and it is an opportunity to learn. During the medical visit, several operators (including residents, senior physicians, deputy head doctors, nurses and 'consultants' (i.e. specialised doctors from other units) pool together their information, knowledge and competences; and thoroughly examine the patient's parameters. Based on all these observations, they build a rational and shared explanation of the perceived clinical behaviour of the patient. The robustness of this process is based on the diversity of their expertise and experiences, as well as on the interaction they have with patients. By virtue of their direct and constant contact with patients, nurses usually feed back a number of signals about patients' conditions that can complete or even modify the diagnosis. The medical visit can be compared to a process of sensemaking (Weick, 1995), which aids the proper reaction when faced with a situation at a given time, and anticipates which future actions to take, as well as the probable risks and adapted countermeasures. By imagining various possible trajectories and complications, doctors suggest alerting signals and control values, and provide instructions for recovery that vary according to the situation, thus allowing nurses to be reactive in case such a problem occurs.

The medical visit usually proceeds smoothly during nominal situations. However, with complex cases, when patients show rare pathologies and there is a lack of literature on the matter, DIY actions and decisions are attempted. Doctors call upon a mix of their theoretical knowledge, previous empirical cases and their intuition. They find subsidiary strategies supported by adapted or invented treatments, assuming that it might be necessary to give up certain care quality criteria, i.e. take greater risks. Again, sacrificing decisions may be taken in such situations (e.g., temporary decrease in the quality of care, decrease of overall patient safety), deviations from the protocol may be made (e.g., disregard of extubation deadlines) or functional reconfigurations are enabled (e.g., a nurse playing the role of a resident). The collective sharing process imposed by the medical visit across the *diversity* of individual perspectives allows staff to limit the associated risk to an acceptable level, based on the *collective consensus*, and to share responsibility among the group.

From Normal Situations to Crisis Management

There is little continuity between the nominal and the crisis functioning modes. There is not only an increase of rhythm, intensity or mobilisation, but also a qualitative rather than quantitative shift: the situation's steering logic changes, priorities, objectives and trade-off criteria are modified, and teams, roles and responsibilities are being reconfigured. More important than the availability of suitable crisis responses, the resilience critical point relies unerringly on *the ability to acknowledge the need to shift* from one mode to the other.

The crisis response is also different in the case of a capacity crisis or in the case of a complexity crisis. In the former case, as already stated, the response basically starts with an over-mobilisation at the bottom of the pyramid. In the latter case, the response basically starts with an over-mobilisation at the top of the pyramid upon the call of seniors and experts from other units, with junior staff (e.g., residents) possibly sidelined, and delegated to 'inferior' tasks.

Coopetition[5] as a Resilience Factor

Until now, we have described rather traditional dimensions of teamwork contributing to the care process resilience. However, complementary and more complex components of the team resilience became apparent during the study. When the patient's condition dynamic accelerates, i.e., when an emergency occurs, and when the intervention speed takes priority, the relationship with protocols is modified. Protocols exist and are necessary, especially for emergencies, but they may need to be adapted – sometimes invented – to have a quicker and more efficient effect. Senior physicians can decide on actions that diverge from the state-of-the-art, and thus allow for a temporarily 'deviant' situation, which is still complying with the unit's ethics. However, because they are not themselves in charge of the implementation of such decisions, doctors need to convince the nurses who actually perform the caring duties. This provides a mechanism of control and mitigation against potential excess. The asymmetry

5 Coopetition, a merging of cooperation and competition, is a neologism coined to describe cooperative competition. Basic principles of coopetitive structures have been described in game theory, a scientific field that received more attention with the book, *Theory of Games and Economic Behavior*, in 1944 and the works of John Forbes Nash on non-cooperative games.

between job profiles is evident. These inventive strategies are rewarding for doctors, demonstrating their autonomy and skills, and produce peers' acknowledgement if successful. However, they put nurses in a risky situation by making them perform outside the protocol's protective scope, by making them directly confront directly the uncertainty of the outcome while in direct contact with the patient, without enabling them to provide the theoretical justification a doctor would be able to give. Thus, it is essential for doctors to explain, convince and make the decision approval an acceptable compromise on behalf of the shared values and acceptable risks. Hence, nurses' resistance can prevent deviations from the state-of-the-art rules. What we have here is an illustration of the benefits, for the system's resilience, of the 'coopetition' between different job profiles. The guiding mechanism of the work group's 'reasonable audacity' towards deviations emerges from this mix of cooperation and competition, and from the diversity of interests.

Similarly, the high level consensus on shared values that can be acknowledged has not inhibited ethical difficulties (a sacrifice remains a sacrifice), nor have the negotiations and conflicts between job profiles. In fact, interests differ when a patient is admitted. For example, one entry means an additional workload for nurses and auxiliary staff, who consequently need to prepare the capacity (bring the required equipment, clean the cubicle). For doctors, a new entry has clinical interest; it is an intellectual stimulus, a challenge or a relevant research opportunity. Again, we have here an illustration of the benefits for the system's resilience of the 'coopetition' between different job profiles. The diversity of interests and the potential for conflict between these different interests reinforces staff adherence to the shared, higher level principles.

Designing Organisational Flexibility: The Question of Front Line Autonomy

Among all the complex reasons that may explain the surprising performance of the HUG– ICU after the merger, we identified the key role of the senior physicians. They are the doctors who lead the daily care operations, and make the medical decisions related to entries, discharges, and therapeutic plans in interaction with the consultants from the different floors within the hospital.

During the crisis merger period, they felt poorly supported and protected in their jobs by the unit management, due to a lack of clarity and poor stability of the framework of policies. They were more directly exposed to the multiple pressures coming from the other hospital units about entries or exits. They were also more directly exposed to the game of power relations between different staff categories, such as doctors and nurses. But at the same time, they benefited from large amounts of autonomy and used it.

For reasons that have not really been explained, and which may well include random factors such as circumstantial personality fit, the senior physicians did not use that autonomy to develop their own idiosyncratic practices but rather they developed a strong team spirit, self-organised themselves, and formed a cohesive group generating a guidance framework that had not been provided by the management. They progressively created new procedural responses and cooperation modes to handle different kinds of situations, particularly degraded or crisis situations. By demonstrating their efficiency, these practices have been maintained over time, taught and distributed throughout the unit. Although it is hard to delineate what part of the resilience demonstrated by the merged ICU is attributable to these measures, this self-organisation does seem to have played a significant positive role. This resonates well with the notion that poly-centric governance is better adapted to generate resilience capacities, at least within an organisation exposed to a high level of uncertainty, such as this ICU.

It is important to note that this self-organisation did not develop against the management. Indeed, while the managers as a team probably allowed their staff more autonomy than intended due to a lack of cohesion, some of them at least – including the head – were concerned about the restoration and maintenance of a common framework amid the turbulence encountered during the merger. They built on the senior physicians' initiatives to endorse and authorise a flexible but shared framework within a process of genuinely normalising positive deviance.

The managers also complemented classical managerial leadership mechanisms by undertaking a comprehensive collective reflection / training approach inspired by the Team Resource Management (TRM) training principles used by the aviation industry. This initiative, called CHLOE (Chemin et al., 2010), was launched in 2008 and involved all the operational care staff (doctors, nurses, aides), including the managers, and has been continued since then. This initiative helped to formulate and disseminate a consensus within the unit about the values that would guide activities. A high- level principle, which was called the 'distributive justice concept', stated that any patient whose clinical state deserves intensive care processes (i.e., would both need it and benefit from it) should be admitted. This meant that someone else had to be discharged if the unit was full, and this led to the powerful patient flow management system described previously. Senior physicians developed a high degree of adherence to that goal, which generated strong solidarity among them.

The Role of Individual Commitment

The daily shocks and constraints of the ICU system cascades down to the operators in the form of contradictory objectives, paradoxical orders and 'hindered quality' (Clot, 2011). This incurs a significant cost, including a cognitive toll, because it assumes alertness and constant focus, and an emotional cost, considering the necessary waiver of certain performance criteria. These costs can be reduced, thanks to unit solidarity, individual and collective competences, agreed protocols, common values backed up by the management, and society's acknowledgement of the importance of this endeavour. However, they are only partly mitigated (Lallement et al., 2011).

Today, resilience in ICUs cannot be separated from a commitment to high levels of individual staff investment, as well as levels of chronic stress that manifests itself in the frequent and significant exhaustion of operators (i.e., burn out). Will it be possible to maintain the performance and resilience of the organisation by slowing down its metabolism? As seen herein, a lot of things have already been done in this direction, intentionally or not. Nevertheless, this study suggests additional leads to achieve further gains. It has shown the fundamental role of reconfiguration, of flexible delegation, of the adaptation of protocols and finally, of trust. This invites a more explicit acknowledgement of these organisational abilities, a finer understanding of their operating modes, and above all, the implementation of specific recurrent training to minimise the stress toll paid by staff. The recent developments and cost decrease in health care simulators, as well as the development of dedicated 'serious games', should be an opportunity to implement a recurrent practice of the corresponding non-technical skills.

Conclusion

Most of the resilience features as described by the resilience engineering theory could be easily observed in this case study. But they had not intentionally been engineered into the ICU; rather they rather emerged from experience. They were facilitated by the self-organisational processes that developed through the organisational crisis following the merger, and were accompanied, but not led, by the management of the unit. Could they be more intentionally engineered (without the support of a crisis)? We believe the answer is yes, and we have started to develop an expanded version of Tables 7.1 and 7.2, that may be used as guidance material for this purpose, for benefits of the ICUs and elsewhere.

Acknowledgements

Our sincere gratitude goes to the Geneva University Hospitals and all the ICU operators who made this research possible, thanks to their availability, their openness to the study and their active participation.

Chapter 8
Investigating Expertise, Flexibility and Resilience in Socio-technical Environments: A Case Study in Robotic Surgery

Anne-Sophie Nyssen and Adélaïde Blavier

Introduction

New technologies in health care are in constant and considerable evolution. They often constitute a type of change implying new knowledge, new skills, but also new work strategies. These recent demands are rarely assessed before the introduction of the technology. It is not unusual for an organisation to rely on medical staff to deal with the technical changes and to adapt their practices in order to keep the level of performance and safety. Because of the rapid advancement of technological development, the capacity to switch smoothly from one technique to another is key to promoting system resilience.

Indeed, several authors have attempted to operationalise the concept of resilience in the real world using the idea of flexibility that reflects the system's capacity to reorient its strategies in order to cope with uncertainty (Hollnagel et al., 2006). Flexibility and adaptivity have often been used as synonymous in scientific literature. Yet, the term 'flexibility' is primarily used to refer to the capacity to switch from one strategy to another, whereas the term 'adaptivity' deals with the capacity to select the most appropriate strategy (Feltovich et al., 1997; Baroody and Rosu, 2006).

A common characteristic of the most renowned disasters such as Chernobyl, Three Mile Island or, more recently, the Air France crash and of the lesser-known accidents in risk systems involved highly experienced operators who continued to persevere on one course of action, despite clear indications that the original assessment was inappropriate. Previously, we have illustrated the dramatic consequences that can have 'perseveration' errors in health care, and showed its propagation over time and space across the medical staff, reproducing the same diagnostic error at different scale levels (individual, team, hospital and network of hospitals) (Nyssen, 2007). A major challenge, thus, for system safety, is to recognise that complex systems are dynamic and to identify the conditions that stimulate adaptivity and strategy flexibility.

The meaningfulness of flexibility / inflexibility is a key element in Hatano's distinction between adaptive–creative and routine–reproductive experts (Hatano, 1982). The experts are adaptive and creative in the sense that they can modify a procedure according to the situation's constraints and invent new strategies when none of the known procedures are effective. In contrast, the routine experts rely on algorithmic procedures, reproducing strategies by which the skills can be performed more accurately and rapidly. However, they are perceived as lacking flexibility in new situations; being able to make only minor adjustments to the procedure, relying on trial and error when confronted with a novel type of problem. The source of flexibility and adaptive expertise seems to rely on a deep conceptual knowledge of the problem at hand that makes it possible to go beyond the powerful influence of the routines and stimulates a switch in strategy according to the unforeseen variability. The distinction between the two types of expertise is largely hypothetical. However, several researchers have recently supported this idea by examples from mathematics education or hypermedia design (Verschaffel et al., 2009, Syer et al., 2003). Further, the distinction does not imply that there are only two categories of expertise. Rather, the acquisition of expertise is referred to as a continuous process and people's position along this continuum can shift as a result of task conditions or personality factors. Better understanding of how expertise is sensitive to uncertainty over time will help us to better appreciate the relationship between flexibility and resilience. This, in turn, will help us to reconsider, if necessary, our safety approach in order to cultivate adaptive–creative expertise and not only routine–reproductive expertise in complex systems.

The path towards adaptive expertise might be different, and even in opposition, to the path towards routine expertise that is acquired through repeated practice in a standardised context. Hatano and Inagaki (1984) have suggested that the socio-cultural context may influence the acquisition of adaptive expertise. The more the system is constrained, the more the work conditions are standardised, the less people will encounter novel problems, the less the need to adjust their skills and the less they will have the opportunity to discuss their performance and to acquire new related conceptual knowledge.

Taking a similar perspective, Pariès (2012) has recently suggested that the usual factors that lead to safety such as normalisation, procedures and standardisation might indeed impair the development of the system's resilience capabilities.

If we can support this idea empirically, it may have a strong impact on training, design and the management of safety programs. In what follows, we refer to a series of illustrative studies to test this hypothesis. In recent years, we were able to observe the introduction of robotic surgery in operating rooms and to study how surgeons adapt their work to continue to perform safely. We were also able to conduct different experimental studies in order to understand better the cognitive processes underlying the acquisition of adaptive expertise.

The Robot–Surgeon System

The robotic surgery was designed in order to recover the 3-D visualisation of the operative field and the degrees of instrument movement freedom lost in classical laparoscopy. The robot system (Da Vinci) consists of two primary components: the surgeon's viewing and control console, and a moveable cart with three articulated robot arms. The surgeon is seated in front of the console, looking at an enlarged three-dimensional binocular display on the operative field while manipulating handles that are similar to joysticks. Manipulation of the handles transmits the electronic signals to the computer that transfers the exact same motions to the robotic arms.

The computer interface has the capability to control and modify the movements of the instrument tips by downscaling deflections at the handles. It can also eliminate physiologic tremor, and adjust grip strength applied to the tools. The computer-generated electrical impulses are transmitted by a 10-metre long cable and command the three articulated 'robot' arms. Disposable laparoscopic articulated instruments are attached to the distal part of two of these arms. The third arm carries an endoscope with dual optical channels, one for each of the surgeon's eyes.

Method

We used the analysis of communication between surgeons as a sign of adaptive capacity. Several studies have focused on the relationship between communication, regular interaction and adaptation and showed both a reduction of verbal information as practitioners get to know each other and an increase of verbal communication during unfamiliar situations or crisis situations (Savoyant and Leplat, 1983; Nyssen and Javaux, 1996; Bressole et al., 1996). In this perspective, changes in verbal communication within an usual team would be the signature of an internal critical state that, in turn, would reveal the system's resilience capacity. The concept of resilience is not new in medical literature. Traditionally, resilience refers to the individual's ability to recover from stresses. More recently, it has been used at a system level as a measure of the system's ability to absorb external changes and stresses while maintaining its functioning and sustainability (Adger et al., 2002; Hollnagel, op. cit.). If the system is dynamic, as we stated before, the resilience ability of the system must be relative and may change over time as underlying components (material or people) and constraints change. In the following examples, we attempt to grasp some of this dynamics, showing how technological changes move the system towards more or less resilience.

We recorded all the verbal communication between the surgeon and the surgeon's assistant. We analysed their content and identified seven categories. We also measured the duration of the intervention, as this is an important performance criterion for surgeons.

The seven categories of communication are:

1. verbal demands concerning the orientation and localisation of organs;
2. verbal demands concerning the manipulation of instruments and / or organs;
3. explicit clarification concerning strategies, plans and procedures;
4. orders referring to tasks such as cutting, changing instruments, and cleaning the camera;
5. explicit confirmation of detection or action;
6. communication referring to state of stress;
7. communication referring to state of relaxation.

In each of the following paragraphs, we consider a critical question about the resilience of socio-technical systems and the answers that our study suggests.

Is the Socio-technical System Resilient to Technological Changes?

Our goal was to study how the system adapts itself to a technological change and if it does, what is the price paid for the resulting resilience? We compared surgical operations that were performed with a robotic system with classical laparoscopy. In the two conditions (robotic and classical laparoscopy), the surgical procedures and the team members were identical. The surgeons were experts in the use of classical laparoscopy (>100 interventions) and were familiar with the use of a robotic system (>10 interventions). We chose two types of surgical procedures (digestive and urological surgery) because it is possible to perform them with either classical laparoscopy or with a robotic system. We observed five cholecystectomies (digestive) using the robotic system and four using classical laparoscopy, and seven prostatectomies (urological) using the robotic system and four using classical laparoscopy. The average duration of the intervention was significantly longer ($p<0.05$) with the robotic system than with classical laparoscopy.

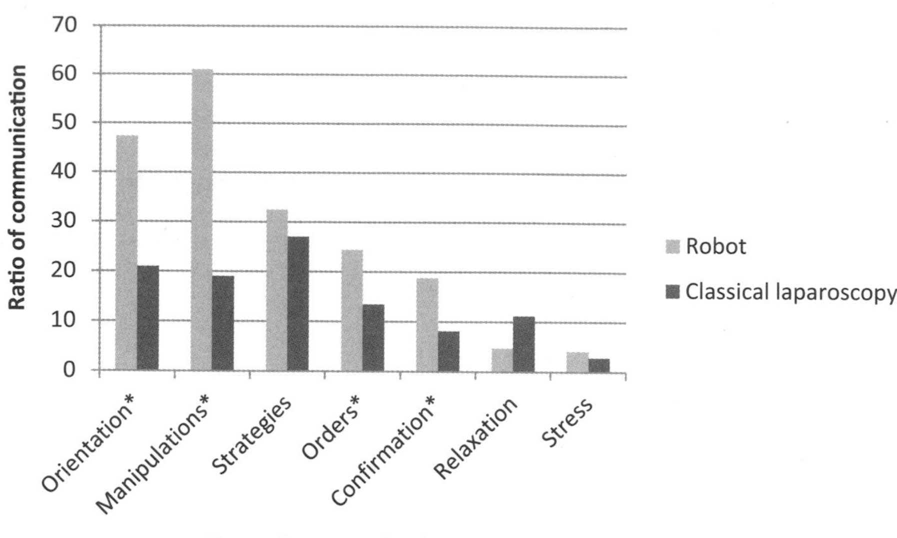

Figure 8.1 Comparison of the communication between robotic and classical laparoscopy

Figure 8.1 shows that the introduction of the robotic system created a new pattern of communication. Our results indicate that not only were there more acts of communication with the robotic system, but also that different types of communication between the surgeon and the assistant were used. This pattern of results was similar for the two types of surgery.

The significant increase in the number of communication acts ($p<0.05$) referring to orientation, manipulation, order and confirmation within the robot system suggests that a breakdown occurs in the collaboration between the surgeons. The robot introduced a distance between the surgeon and the assistant that impedes face-to-face, implicit communication and prevents the assistant from anticipating; the surgeon then continually needs to ask the assistant about the orientation and the placement of the instrument (which is manipulated by him) in order to facilitate the identification of the organs. Therefore, it seems clear that the robot changes the feedback loop and that verbal communication used by surgeons is an adaptive process to compensate the loss of face-to-face feedback, absent in the robotic configuration. The socio-technical system here can be considered relatively resilient to technological change but resilience comes at the cost of requiring more explicit communication from the members of the team that is time and resource consuming and, in some ways, 'unnatural' in terms of adaptation process for the team.

Is the Socio-technical System Resilient to Surprises?

During our study we observed four emergency conversion decisions i.e, to switch from robot surgery to classical surgery: two in cardiology during our pre-observations and two during our experimental study, one in urology and one in digestive surgery. Each conversion required a switch of strategy from robotic to laparoscopic or open surgery (digestive surgery to laparoscopic surgery and cardiac surgery to open surgery). These switches of strategy imply an instrumental switch and sometimes a perceptive switch (from 3-D to 2-D, from robotic to laparoscopic).

We observed that each conversion is associated with an increased number of verbal communications (Figure 8.2). These communications concerned stress, explicit clarification of strategies (re-planning) and expectations concerning orientation and manipulations. We also observed less communication referring to confirmation. During a crisis, the surgeon does not take the time to verify the receipt of his action or request. This pattern of verbal communication reveals a critical internal state and an 'emergency adaptation' process. Conversion decisions were taken when confronted with a patient presenting an 'anomaly' of anatomy. In this sense, we can consider that the robot–surgeons system is vulnerable to unforeseen variability that falls outside the designer's model of a 'universal' patient.

In each case, we observed that the surgeon had the ability to switch to appropriate alternative strategies using another human–machine system such as open or laparoscopy techniques, relying on his experience and knowledge with this system. These examples indicate that resilience here lies in the strategic flexibility of experts, rather than in their speed and accuracy of routine skills.

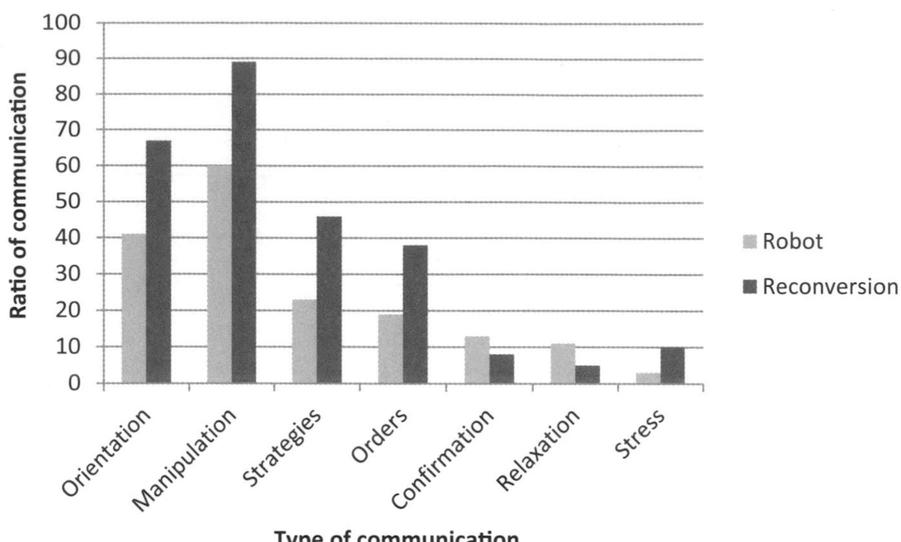

Figure 8.2 **Type and frequency of communication during reconversion**

How Does Learning Context Hamper or Facilitate Adaptive-flexibility Expertise in the Example System?

The acquisition of expertise is undoubtedly based upon the accumulation of experience within an environment. Routine skills are useful as long as this environment is constant (i.e. the same set of devices (and people) is available. In health care, although resources such as equipment or expertise are limited because of economical and qualification considerations, innovations are constantly introduced that require new skills and new knowledge. So, there is a great need for generating adaptive–creative expertise.

Forty medical students without any surgical experience were randomised into four groups (classical laparoscopy with 3-D direct view or with 2-D indirect view, robotic system in 3-D or in 2-D) and repeated a task six times. The task involved passing, in succession, a needle with a thread attached through rings placed at different heights and depths. The 'rings' routes required a lot of the usual fine movements required in minimal invasive surgery (grasping a needle, curving and introducing it, etc.).

After six repetitions, they performed two trials with the same technique but in the other viewing condition (perceptive switch);

then they performed the last three trials with the technique they never used (technical switch). For each trial, we calculated a performance score based on the number of rings which the subjects went through with the needle in four minutes. All procedures were video-recorded and accuracy was evaluated by three independent observers (Blavier et al., 2007).

Performance of all subjects improved from their first to sixth trial ($F(5,180) = 25.52$, $P. < 0.000$), but learning curves were significantly different according to the technique and the viewing conditions ($F(15,180) = 2.12$, $P < 0.005$). The 3-D view (classical and robotic laparoscopy) facilitated a substantial, rapid improvement, whereas the improvement was very weak for classical laparoscopy with 2-D-indirect view.

Perceptive Switch (after Trial 6)

After the perceptive switch (Figure 8.3), as expected, subjects' performance was affected by the 2-D to 3-D change. In the two trials of this phase, the performance was only differentiated by the perceptive dimension, with better performance in 3-D view (classical and robotic system) than in 2-D view. Furthermore, performance was stable without any positive or negative evolution during the two trials.

Instrumental Switch (after Trial 8)

After the technical switch (Figure 8.4), the performance in all conditions decreased to the same score as in the first trial. Moreover, the performance did not much improve in this final phase. Participants showed difficulty adapting their movements to the other technique: with the robotic system, subjects kept a conservative strategy used in classical laparoscopy and showed difficulty moving the camera, and with classical laparoscopy, manipulation of long and rigid instruments seemed to be the most difficult obstacle to overcome. However, the improvement and best performance in the last trial in classical laparoscopy with a direct view showed that the 3-D view allowed efficient overlap of instrumental difficulty in classical laparoscopy (for a complete description of this study, see Blavier et al., 2007).

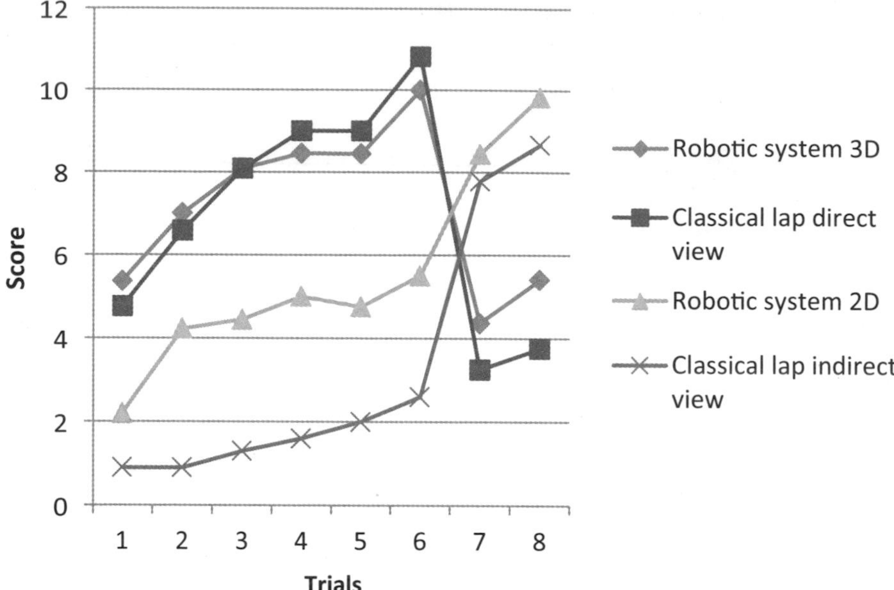

Figure 8.3 Perceptive switch

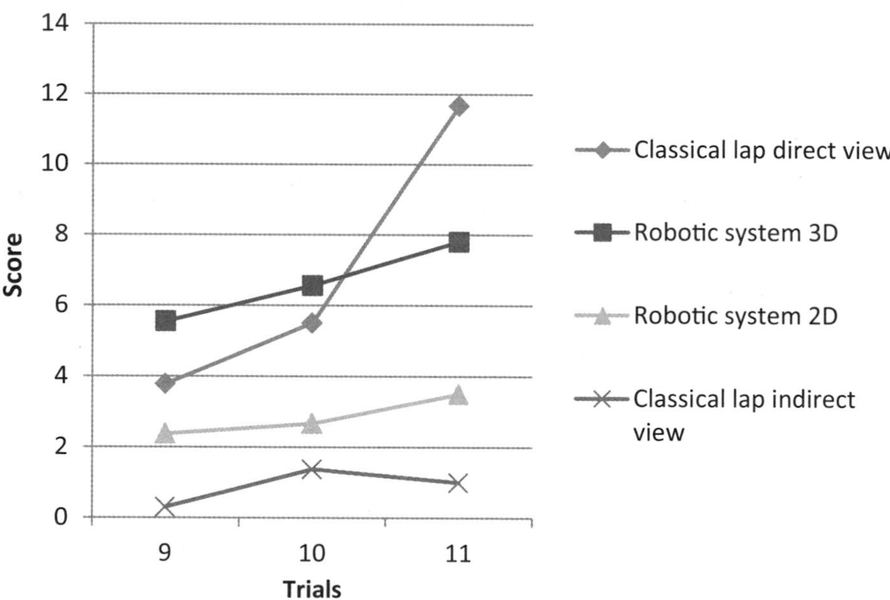

Figure 8.4 Instrumental switch

These data provide us some information about the impact of the learning context on the development of adaptive skills. They suggest that adaptive expertise may not simply come with time and that the path to developing adaptive-flexible or routine-inflexible expertise may be influenced by the socio-technical in which skills are learned.

Discussion

Up to now, safety has been improved using technology developments, standardisation, protocols and training. In this approach, the focus is on the 'causal factor', concentrated on the cause of the accident, classified as either a technical or human cause. This approach has significantly improved safety in many complex domains, including health care. For example, in anaesthesia the risk of death as a result of general anaesthesia has decreased over the past 20 years from 1/1,000 to 1/100,000 acts thanks to the development of devices, drugs and standards. However, in recent years, even if safety continues to improve, it seems that traditional safety tools will fail to reduce the residual components of accidents. Moreover, it appears that traditional safety tools contribute, to some extent, to the complexity of the system, increasing the risk of error or deviation.

A complementary approach is the resilience engineering approach, or Safety-II approach, in Hollnagel's terminology. Here, attention is paid to the system's abilities to perform and to succeed in varying situations including under technological change. Activity analysis in context has been the pillar of the French-speaking ergonomic approach. In 1967, Faverge (1979) had already highlighted the need to describe the regulation process used in the daily work activity to cope with variability and uncertainty. Research on human reliability has progressively shifted the focus of attention from the spectrum of work activity (with and without error) to the much smaller component of safety associated to errors and failures of adaptation, thus forgetting that 'correct performance and systematic errors are two sides of the same coin' (Reason, 1990).

Using different illustrative studies, we wanted in this chapter to focus understanding on how a socio-technical system adapts itself to change and uncertainty in order to address key training, design and management safety considerations.

The first two studies based upon field observations show that the system's resilience ability comes at the cost of changing cooperation modes and increasing the need for verbal communication between the members of the team. We first demonstrated that the system can be considered resilient to technological change and that it experiences from the benefits of technology. The robot interface improves the quality of the surgery by eliminating the surgeon's tremor and downscaling the deflection at handles. However, at the same time, the robot increases the total time taken in the surgical procedure and modifies the structure of the team, creating brittleness with respect to the need for cooperation. So, if resilience can be observed at the system level, the assessment may be different at the team and individual levels over time, when the consequences of the technological change will be felt. The surgeon is isolated from the rest of the team. The surgeon's assistant becomes more like a technician, responding to the orders of the surgeon and there is a new player who becomes essential: the technician. As a result, we can predict that the status of the team members will be modified. This observation highlights the fact that assessment of resilience should be determined at different time and structural scales.

As uncertainty increases due to the unforeseen variability of the patients, initial procedures that are operationalised through preparatory configurations become irrelevant and conversion decisions become imperative. Devices (or protocols) in health care are designed on the basis of models of patients, drugs, problems and users, creating the opportunity of 'anomaly' or exception and, in turn, of conversion. Each of these conversions is associated with an increased number of verbal communications that are needed to clarify, share plans and organise the activity between the surgeons. The conversion cases represent a fundamental breakdown of the system, yet we have seen how the surgeons, and not the robot, have the resources for handling the event before it affects the patient by shifting from the robotic procedure to a classical one (open or laparoscopy surgery). This can be done because the 'old' techniques and the corresponding skills are still available in the system.

Thus, the system's resilience emerges through the history and the diversity of agent–environment interactions that enhance the surgeon's autonomy towards the unforeseen constraints of the design. There is no necessity for innovation to cope with uncertainty. Rather, it is the repeated application of the skills in different socio-technical environments that leads to adaptive-creative expertise and allows the surgeon to inhibit perseveration and to switch between strategies in their repertoire. Therefore, it seems clear that the current approach of safety based upon standardisation and protocols encourages routine expertise but militates against adaptive expertise and, in turn, against resilience.

With the third study, we wanted to take our reflections a step further and investigate the training consequences of our findings and the path towards adaptive expertise. Several authors argue that it is best to teach routine expertise and only afterwards change one's training program in the direction of adaptive expertise (Geary, 2003). Others warn against the rigidifying effects of routine practice that may impede the development of adaptive expertise (Feltovitch, et al., 1997; Hatano and Oura, 2003). Using an experimental environment, we were able to compare the impact of different learning activities on adaptive performance. First, we showed a decrease in performance of all subjects (whatever their training program) after both the technical and the perceptive switch, suggesting that there is no transfer of skills from one technique to another. Second, we showed that learning with the robot seems to impair learning with laparoscopic techniques, suggesting that the robot could lead to a relative rigidity in acting and thinking and, in turn, to a reduction in cognitive flexibility. This rigidity effect has not been observed in the direction of laparoscopic to robotic surgery, as our field studies confirmed.

This brings us to a question we have not raised yet but which emerges from the discussion: how to maintain these routine or 'Jurassic' skills to be able to mobilise them when confronted with uncertainty, when and for how long? Should we make mandatory recurrent practice with 'old' technology? Should we use training simulators? More studies are needed to be able to answer these questions and to explore the developmental aspect of adaptive–routine expertise. However, for reasons that we have elaborated through this chapter, we can say that the most valuable instructional approach will not be one wherein the medical staff receives repeated practice in algorithmic techniques for selecting the most efficient strategy, as proposed by many new medical curricula, textbooks and simulator training programs, but rather an approach characterised by an effective balance between routine and adaptive expertise acquisition. This seems to require conditions that cultivate diversity and allow repeated interaction with various socio-technical environments. Since new technology fascinates people, this might not be as easy to promote in health care as in other socio-technical systems.

Acknowledgements

We would like to thank the surgeons who participated in the various studies, and in particular, M.D. Guy-Bernard Cadière for his long-term cooperation.

Chapter 9
Reconciling Regulation and Resilience in Health Care

Carl Macrae

Introduction

Death, taxes – and regulation. Few things in life are certain, but when it comes to animated debates on the organisation and quality of health care systems, these three come close. Regulation is a ubiquitous and expanding feature of modern health care systems, but one that is much maligned by many health care workers. Regulation, in the form of standards, rules, protocols, targets and the like, remains one of the key drivers of the structure of health care activities and the design of health care organisations. Regulation is often one of the first levers that policy makers and professional bodies reach for to drive improvements in quality and safety, or when confronted by concerns about substandard performance. Yet the relationship between regulation and resilience in health care remains little explored, with each set of ideas sometimes posed as unreconcilable to the other. This chapter explores the role of regulation in producing or potentially undermining resilient performance in health care. It argues that the interfaces between regulation and resilience are complex and that the role of regulation in producing resilience in health care is often under-appreciated, but nonetheless critical.

At core, regulation can be defined as a systematic attempt to shape, monitor, control and modify practices and technologies within organisations in order to achieve some desired state of affairs (Hutter, 2001). In health care, this usually involves a central agency, such as the Care Quality Commission in

England, setting, monitoring and enforcing specific standards across a range of health care providers. Often these regulatory requirements become embedded in the practice of health care organisations in the form of formal standards, specified rules, predefined protocols and prescribed processes that are put in place to constrain action, optimise performance and prevent error. These forms of organisational prediction and control form the basis of most regulatory regimes, but seem to fly in the face of the basic tenets of thinking on resilience. Resilience broadly refers to an organisation's ability to contain adaptively, correct and respond to disruptions before these disable their operations and cause serious breakdowns (Collingridge, 1996; Weick et al., 1999; Hollnagel et al., 2008; Hollnagel et al., 2010). The organisational capabilities that provide resilience are usually understood as dependent on decentralised, improvised, adaptive and flexible processes that creatively make use of the local resources and the emergent expertise present in any particular situation (Hollnagel et al., 2006; Comfort, Boin and Demchak, 2010).

Not only do the basic mechanisms of regulation therefore appear at odds with ideas of resilience but the very notion of regulation and regulators can often provoke considerable antipathy amongst health care workers. Many associate the idea of regulation with externally imposed, bureaucratic, heavy-handed, burdensome, box-ticking exercises that distract them from the real work of caring for patients – and that is putting it politely. A few hours spent on a typical hospital ward is enough to appreciate where this view of regulation might come from. Protocols, policies, checklists, standards, guidelines, pathways, reporting, audits, data returns: there are certainly more than enough of these to go around. And with increasing pressures for standardisation and accountability in health care, the trend only appears to be heading in one direction. Those working at the sharp end of health care may be forgiven for feeling awash in regulation at times.

Yet, speak to patients and you might hear quite a different story, particularly from those who have been on the receiving end of poor quality care – or from the relatives who survive them. In this view, health care regulation is too soft, regulators are not intrusive enough, and controls, monitoring and enforcement need to be increased to stop bad things happening again – views that routinely surface after major health care scandals, such as the enquiry into failures of care at the Mid Staffordshire Foundation Trust in the English NHS (Golding, 2012). There can be truth in both of these positions – that there is both too much and not enough regulation in health care. The devil is, of course, in the detail. Depending on how specific regulatory tools are designed, implemented and responded to, regulation might be a powerful force for improvement or it might be a wasteful distraction.

It is understandable that the topic of health care regulation is often subject to both emotive and polarised debate, both in popular and professional discourse, as well as in more theoretical arenas. It is a topic that can at times be tainted by politics, polemic, prejudices and personal frustrations. This is a shame, particularly because the role of regulation in supporting resilience is an important but nuanced one – and nuance is often the first casualty of politics. This chapter explores a more subtle view on regulation and some of its key points of intersection with the ideas – and ideals – of resilience. First, the basic mechanics of regulation and resilience are introduced and compared, with the suggestion that the processes involved in each are not as far removed as they may first appear. Then, two key interfaces of regulation and resilience in health care are examined: standardisation and centralisation. These are two frequent flash-points in debates regarding the expansion of regulation in health care that are often simplified in binary terms that contrast the standardisation produced by many forms of regulation with the flexibility demanded for resilience, pitching the centralising tendencies of regulation against the decentralisation required for resilient performance. A more nuanced analysis can reveal subtle and important interactions between mechanisms of regulation and those of resilience. Understanding these interactions is essential to designing regulatory regimes that support safe, high-quality and resilient health care.

Understanding Regulation and Resilience

The ultimate objective of health care regulation is to improve performance and to reduce risk (Walshe, 2003). Likewise, resilience is posited as an organisational capability that can support high levels of performance and safety (Sutcliffe and Vogus, 2003). Yet the ideas and literatures that underpin each of these approaches to health care improvement rarely come into direct contact. In fact, regulation in its various forms is often held up as representing the antithesis of resilience. Regulation is commonly understood to depend on anticipatory rules, structures, plans, routines and protocols that are at odds with the in-the-moment adaptive, mindful and flexible capacities that are seen as the basis of resilience. These seemingly simple distinctions can break down on closer inspection. When viewed at the level of organisational practices, the activities and work that are involved in regulating risk and responding resiliently can look quite similar. Both depend to a large degree on those working on the front line of health care organisations: just as resilient performance results from the engagement of a wide array of staff in safety improvement, so regulation is a broad and pervasive activity. 'Regulatory work' is not simply within the remit of staff with specific roles such as risk manager or compliance officer, but is done by nurses coordinating care pathways, surgeons completing checklists, infection control specialists organising hand washing campaigns and health care assistants submitting patient safety incident reports. Regulatory work takes many forms and is widely distributed across organisations. At core, the practices that both produce resilience and regulate performance are those that are focused on continually formalising, monitoring and improving organisational practices – iterative processes in which current practices are observed, reflected on and continually adapted (Macrae, 2010).

At a more general level of description, commonalities are equally apparent. The basic functions of regulation depend on a recursive process of gathering information about organisational performance, setting standards and monitoring for deviance, and then modifying and altering behaviour as required (Hood et al., 2001). The social-cognitive processes of resilience appear equally to depend on attentive and mindful engagement with organisational activities, continual monitoring for deviations from expectations, and responding to disruptions by adapting and altering activities (Weick et al., 1999). Both functionally and in practice, regulatory work and resilient performance can be hard to unpick neatly.

Despite apparent commonalities at both a general level of description and at the level of situated practice, the infrastructures and technologies that enact regulation typically appear radically different from specific prescriptions for resilience that include responding creatively and adapting to emerging situations. This is most evident in the profusion of clinical guidelines, quality standards, policies, protocols and procedures that are increasingly being produced in health care. These are all technologies that seek to constrain, predetermine and delimit the scope of acceptable action in a given situation. They are often employed as tools that allow a centralised authority to standardise, supervise and control local action at a distance (Woods and Shattuck, 2000). It is here, in the ways that regulatory technologies of control are designed and implemented, that the most striking distinctions between resilience and regulation become apparent. Regulatory technologies that aim to support centralised and standardised control of behaviour appear immediately at odds with the emphasis that most models of resilience place on local innovations, flexibility, improvisation, adaptability, problem solving, vigilance and trial-and-error learning (Wildavksy, 1988; Bigley and Roberts, 2001; Hollnagel et al., 2006; Reason, 1997). While definitions of resilience often remain purposefully broad, encompassing a range of organisational capabilities, the core principles focus on the importance of locally produced innovations to resolve locally encountered problems, and on the capacity for individuals to organise flexibly and adaptably in the face of unexpected events. These ideals of resilience emphasise the value of decentralised and distributed authority that allows professional judgement and expert discretion, particularly in the face of high levels of variability, uncertainty and change: characteristics that are all present in abundance in many domains of health care, and that traditional regulatory tools can be ill-equipped to handle.

Many of the challenges and criticisms associated with regulation relate equally to the proliferation, misdirection and impracticality of the design and implementation of many specific regulatory tools – and the inadvertent consequences this poor design can bring. Regulation is a serious business and stakes can be high. For instance, in England, the Care Quality Commission (CQC) sets a range of quality standards for health care providers, monitors and inspects providers in relation to those standards, and takes enforcement action in cases where those standards have been breached – up to and including cancelling a provider's registration: essentially removing their permit to operate. Similarly, in the USA, the Joint Commission for Accreditation of Health Care Organisations routinely inspects hospitals to ensure that a variety of standards are being met, with accreditation being critical to a hospital retaining its license in many states. With this much riding on compliance, organisations can become overly focused on meeting regulatory requirements merely to manage the risks of regulatory sanctions (Brennan and Berwick, 1996), at the expense of actually managing the underlying risks to quality and safety that the regulations are intended to address – so called 'secondary risk management' (Power, 2007). Further, as most major health care systems are supervised by a range of regulatory agencies, there can be a complex network of regulatory requirements to navigate, produced by statutory regulators, professional associations, national agencies, non-governmental organisations, insurers, commissioners and many other organisations. There may be few pressures within a system of regulation to rationalise overlapping or conflicting requirements and tools, as each of these regulators may individually have an incentive to increase the scope of their regulatory remit and territory (Walshe, 2003). Likewise, when standards, requirements and protocols are designed far from the front line, they can become impractical and at times unworkable at the 'sharp end' of organisations (Hutter, 2001) – rendering systems of regulation on paper that bear little relation to actual practices.

Poorly designed and implemented regulation can therefore dramatically reduce the attentional resources, local authority and capacity for flexibility on the front line of health care organisations. That is, poor regulation can reduce organisational capacities for resilience. Moreover, poorly designed regulatory tools can potentially undermine the legitimacy of an entire regulatory regime. These adverse consequences of regulation are often the ones that gain most attention: stories of endless red tape and form filling. The ways in which regulation can support resilience in organisations and across health care systems are discussed less often. Two arenas where regulation can actively support resilience in health care are also two of the most contested, and are examined next. They focus on activities that at first blush appear directly opposed to principles of resilience: standardisation and centralisation.

Standardisation

Standardisation is a key regulatory activity. The history of safety and quality in health care is, to a large extent, the history of standardisation by means of checklists, protocols, training, and design. All of these activities in some way seek to standardise and systematise different elements of health care practice. Yet standardisation still has something of a bad name in health care. It can be seen as undermining the discretion and autonomy of health professionals – and is most vocally met by doctors, who particularly prize their professional autonomy, though all health care workers rely to a large degree on discretion and local decision making to work effectively. For the same reasons, standardisation equally appears to run against basic ideals of resilience. And yet in subtle ways, efforts to standardise activities can be supportive of, and potentially essential to, resilient systems of health care.

One way that standardisation, when applied appropriately, can support resilience is by reducing requirements on health care workers for conscious, effortful attention to trivial details. This can free up attentional capacity from mundane issues, such as working out the unique layout of this particular operating theatre, allowing attention to be allocated to the truly complex and pressing issues, such as working out how to deal with unexpected problems intubating the patient. Standardisation can reduce the trivial uncertainties and variations in the basic systems and processes that health care workers depend upon, freeing up their intellectual resources to focus on the uncertainties and variations that matter. A key assumption here is that individuals and organisations have a finite adaptive capacity available to respond to unexpected events. If this adaptive capacity is continually being depleted by lazy design or organisation-induced variation, then less adaptive capacity remains to deal with patient-induced variation – the variation that actually matters.

Infusion pumps offer a simple example. A typical hospital in the UK will have around 30 different designs of infusion pump. Many of these pumps are so different that even the layout of the numeric keypads are reversed from one model so the next – with either the digit '1' at the top left of the keypad, as is the convention on a mobile phone, or at the bottom left, as is the convention on a calculator. This is an extraordinarily minor variation on an extremely routine piece of equipment. But it begs a fundamental question: is this the sort of variation that health care workers should be expending their limited attentional resources in resolving? And also, if these easy and trivial targets for standardisation have not yet been addressed, what variations in the rest of a hospital's systems and equipment are draining adaptive capacity? Careful standardisation of what should be automatic and routine components of health care work can increase the overall adaptive capacity, and resilience, of a system by reducing distraction and increasing attentional resources for making the challenging decisions and judgements that patient care often requires. Standardisation can provide the stable background against which important fluctuations and variations can be identified. Regulation and resilience can work in the same direction.

Centralisation

Centralisation is a core feature of many regulatory activities in health care. Standards are set and monitored by centralised regulatory agencies. Oversight and supervision is performed through centralised hierarchies, both within health care organisations and across health care systems. The centralisation of authority, information and control appears to run counter to the principles of locally distributed adaptation and trial-and-error learning that characterise resilience (Wildavsky, 1988). Yet in some ways, resilient health care systems can only function with appropriate centralisation – to coordinate and spread lessons from local improvements, and also to help ensure that local adaptations in one area of a system do not adversely impact on other areas of the system (Woods and Branlat, 2011a).

A clear example is provided by safety incident reporting. Adapting locally to unexpected events, and learning from experience and errors, are two defining features of resilience. Patient safety incident reporting systems represent formalised structures to support these activities, and are operated by most health care organisations in advanced economies. Translating the local lessons from incidents into widespread improvements across entire health care systems depends in large part on centralised systems of reporting and communication. Responding to an event locally by changing policies and practice in a particular ward or organisation represents a resilient response for a single organisation. But to ensure resilience across an entire health care system, those lessons and improvements must be spread. This requires drawing on a local lesson and circulating it to other local sites, where that information can be adapted and implemented according to local circumstances. The widespread circulation of local information requires some form of centralised communication or transmission mechanism: a central shared space, or clearing house, that is accessible and connected to a wide range of organisations. This is in much the same way as the social networks of Facebook and Twitter allow the massive sharing of highly local and specific information amongst networks of peers, but this depends on all users of the network pooling and accessing their information through a single, centralised shared space where they all go to interact.

One example of this centralisation of decentralised information in health care – or the regulation of resilience – is provided by a haemodialysis incident that occurred in the National Health Service in 2008, and the mechanisms that the National Reporting and Learning System provided to centralise, review and then spread this information throughout the health care system. One day in September 2008, a single hospital trust encountered an unexpected and serious event: soon after discharge, several haemodialysis patients were readmitted to hospital suffering from acute haemolysis – a dramatic destruction of red blood cells with severe complications. One patient died and four others required blood transfusions (National Patient Safety Agency, 2008). Rapid investigation by the hospital trust identified that silver stabilised hydrogen peroxide had been added to the hospital's main water system to address water quality issues the day before these patients received their haemodialysis treatment. In this hospital, the renal unit took water from the hospital's main water system before filtering and treating it for use in the dialysis systems. On this occasion, the renal unit had not been informed that the hydrogen peroxide treatment was taking place. The various water filters and treatment systems in the renal unit cannot filter out hydrogen peroxide, which passed straight through into the patients' bloodstreams.

In response to this event, national safety alerts were sent out to all health care trusts across the country requiring immediate review of these potential risks. Trusts were required to review systems and adapt and improve processes for notifying and alerting departments of water treatment within 30 days. This was a rapid, centralised response to a local incident. It targeted local improvements on a national scale. The safety alert did not prescribe in detail how organisations needed to respond, only that they should respond. It demonstrates how centralised systems of monitoring, surveillance and communication can capture local lessons and amplify and circulate them across an entire health care system, translating resilience at an organisational level into resilience at the level of an entire health care system – and achieving this through a highly centralised regulatory system. One of the ironies of this story is that that National Patient Safety Agency that coordinated these local responses and others like it has since been abolished by the UK government (Scarpello, 2010), in line with the principle that patient safety should primarily be a local responsibility, and power and authority should be returned to the hands of local clinicians and away from centralised oversight agencies acting at a distance. The role that centralisation plays in supporting local resilience and improvement can be subtle and, indeed, easily ignored.

Conclusion

At first blush, regulation and resilience seem uneasy bedfellows. Regulation and regulatory activities are often viewed quite narrowly in health care. Regulation largely focuses on shaping health care systems through pre-planned, highly specified, centralised and standardised operating models that seek to constrain and delimit acceptable action. Resilience, on the other hand, is typically viewed as the product of locally adaptive, flexible and improvised responses to unexpected events that depend on professional discretion and local expertise. However, rather than binary opposites, or even opposite ends of a spectrum, the interfaces between regulation and resilience are more subtle and nuanced. Regulation can actively support organisational capacities for organisational resilience, and can provide mechanisms and structures through which resilience is generated across entire health care systems.

The points of intersection between these different strategies for improving quality and safety are complex and multifarious. They need closer examination and explanation, preferably at the level of the situated practices and organisational mechanisms that produce them. These relationships also beg a question of resilience itself. If resilience can be supported and amplified through careful regulatory design, to what extent can regulation itself become resilient? How can health care implement mechanisms that allow locally derived improvements and lessons to be incorporated back into national policy and regulatory processes? By tackling these questions and improving the resilience of health care and its regulatory regimes, we can hope to reduce the other unfortunate certainties of health care: avoidable patient harm and death, and their heavy burden on patients, families – and taxpayers.

Acknowledgements

This work was kindly supported by the Health Foundation, an independent charity working continuously to improve the quality of health care in the UK.

Chapter 10
Re-structuring and the Resilient Organisation: Implications for Health Care

Robyn Clay-Williams

Introduction

Restructuring – in response to forces such as government or regulatory authority mandate, technological change, or economic pressure – is a common phenomenon in health care. Both the formal and social structures that make up a health care system regularly change as a result of such reorganisations. While a resilient system is 'able effectively to adjust its functioning prior to, during, or following changes and disturbances, so that it can continue to perform as required after a disruption or major mishap' (Hollnagel, 2009b: 177), much of the research in health care involves change at the level of departments or teams (and centres on form rather than function). At the higher level of health care organisations, change often involves transformation rather than 'elasticity'. Research into socio-ecological resilience explores this phenomenon, where structural changes of sufficient magnitude can result in transformation, rather than maintenance, of function. While they can be abrupt or gradual, these adaptive or generative processes often occur over a longer timescale than the system changes generally addressed by engineering resilience. This chapter presents a theory of adaptive change and resilience derived from the behaviour of large and complex ecosystems, and discusses the implications of this theory for health care restructuring and resilience.

Health Care is a Complex Adaptive System

Health care, as described in Chapter 6, is a complex adaptive system – complex in that there are a large number of interacting services consisting of other services, agents and processes, and adaptive in that the system is able to self-organise and learn. Organisations such as health care can be viewed through a number of different lenses (Bolman and Deal, 2008) and each lens reveals a different picture. One picture is the management structure – the 'wiring diagram' of who reports to whom, and how different departments are interconnected to conduct the 'business' of medical treatment. This is an aggregated view of the organisation. Another picture is the organisational culture or social system – how things are done around here, and how clinicians interact with patients and each other. This is a more fine-grained view of the organisation. Alternately, we can look from a human capability viewpoint: how do people connect, learn and grow from their work? Or we can peer through the political lens to see how power is wielded in the organisation, and how decisions are made. In a more tangible sense, the organisation is also comprised of physical entities – the architecture, layout and location of the buildings, and the associated infrastructure and utilities.

When viewed through a structural lens, hospitals are traditionally a dual hierarchy (Rizzo, House and Lirtzman, 1970), comprising the business activity of managing the hospital and the clinical activity of caring for the patients. These are nested systems with different but interacting objectives and timescales. Within the realm of clinical activity, there are nested systems of professions such as doctor, nurse, or allied health, and within these are nested sub-systems of specialisations, such as cardiac surgeon or pharmacist. Business activities also comprise a number of systems and sub-systems such as administration and finance, human resources, safety and quality, and so on. In addition to hierarchies, there are also simultaneously non-hierarchical, networked or cross-linked relationships. Recent developments have resulted in new organisation-wide structural systems comprising clinical directorates; clinical directorates usually consist of both clinical and management professionals, and are typically structured according to either medical domain, or to body system or type of disease (Braithwaite, 2006).

Adaptive Processes

To examine adaptive processes, we first need to define our system of interest. By defining the boundaries of a system, we can determine whether influences are external or internal (remembering that these assignments are arbitrary, depending on our selected boundary). A problem in health care is that the boundaries can be porous, ill defined and dynamic. The easiest boundaries to define are those of the physical hospital system comprising the buildings, power and utilities, and other infrastructure. This system is 'concrete' and normally changes very slowly, if at all. Perhaps because of the ease in defining this system, the resilience of the physical hospital when disturbed by extreme events – such as storm, power failure, or seismic activity – has been well studied (Carthey, Chandra and Loosemore, 2008; Carthey, Chandra and Loosemore, 2009; Cimellaro, Reinhorn and Bruneau, 2010).

More commonly, we are interested in the provision of the 'function' of delivering health care services, and while for acute care this normally occurs within the physical bounds of the hospital, it can also be provided independently of structural components if necessary. Defining the 'functional' boundary of the health care system is more difficult, as the boundaries change depending on the framework through which they are viewed, and also over time. We cannot easily 'see' this system and it is perhaps easier to define boundaries in terms of what is internal and what is external to the problem under consideration. While internal processes may intuitively seem more relevant to the problem, outside interactions and influences can also be critical to improving system operation and performance.

Complex adaptive systems continually self-replicate and organise to improve their ability to adapt and innovate (Alderson and Doyle, 2010). Evolution is the process of variation, interaction and selection that occurs within systems and sub-systems. Change can be viewed in two ways: the internal dynamics of the evolving system, or externally applied (sometimes mandated) change. Mandated change is often a perturbation that overlies or modulates the natural tendency of the system to evolve. System disturbances (whether mandated or not) can vary in magnitude, pattern and duration. Baseline patterns can be constant, increasing, decreasing, or cyclical. Short-term acute perturbations above baseline – an outbreak of influenza or natural disasters such as floods or cyclones – can occur. Medium- to long-term changes, such as organisation reshuffles, government budgetary adjustments, or new regulations, can also provide positive or adverse influences.

Disturbances can also be characterised, either at the level of events or patterns, according to their predictability. Westrum (2006) terms perturbations that are regular or predictable (whether short, medium or long term) 'regular threats', whereas those perturbations that are random are termed (depending on their magnitude) either 'irregular threats', or 'unexampled threats'. 'Irregular threats' are one-off events that can be managed – with difficulty – whereas 'unexampled threats' are so large or unpredictable that the outcome is catastrophic. Stressors can be internal, external or both. Within a system such as health care, there are multi-layered systems, multiple stressors, multiple equilibria and even continual change. These systems operate in an environment that is constantly changing and there is a complex bidirectional feedback between the systems reacting with each other and their external environment. The interactions with multiple human elements in the system, and the creativity, unpredictability and variability of those elements will also create stabilising and destabilising forces.

To investigate resilience and how it may be characterised in health care, it is useful to look for analogies in other large complex dynamic systems that have been extensively studied. One such system is biology and how life evolves and is sustained in the environment. Gunderson and Holling (2002) explain dynamic ecosystem behaviour in terms of a natural complex adaptive cycle, resulting from the interplay between the potential of the system for change, its degree of connectedness and its resilience (Figure 10.1). Firstly, the potential for change can be thought of in terms of accumulated resources, and connectedness as the sensitivity of system processes to external variation. Connectedness provides additional links, or potential mechanisms to deal with variation, and therefore greater redundancy within the system. So, over time, an immature system will slowly grow (r) and develop increased connections and accumulate resources. It will eventually reach a point where the tightness of coupling within the system will make it fragile (K) and failure will occur (Ω). Failure releases the energy bound in the system, and frees resources for reorganisation to take place (α). There is maximum potential for system learning or adaptation to occur at this point. Depending on the nature of the reorganisation, the system then repeats the cycle, or transforms to a new type of system. In ecosystems, we see an adaptive cycle of exploitation, conservation, creative destruction and renewal that occurs at various levels within a system and at various rates. Crises result in additional emergent functionality and processes, and there is greater interaction between processes and the environment in order to survive.

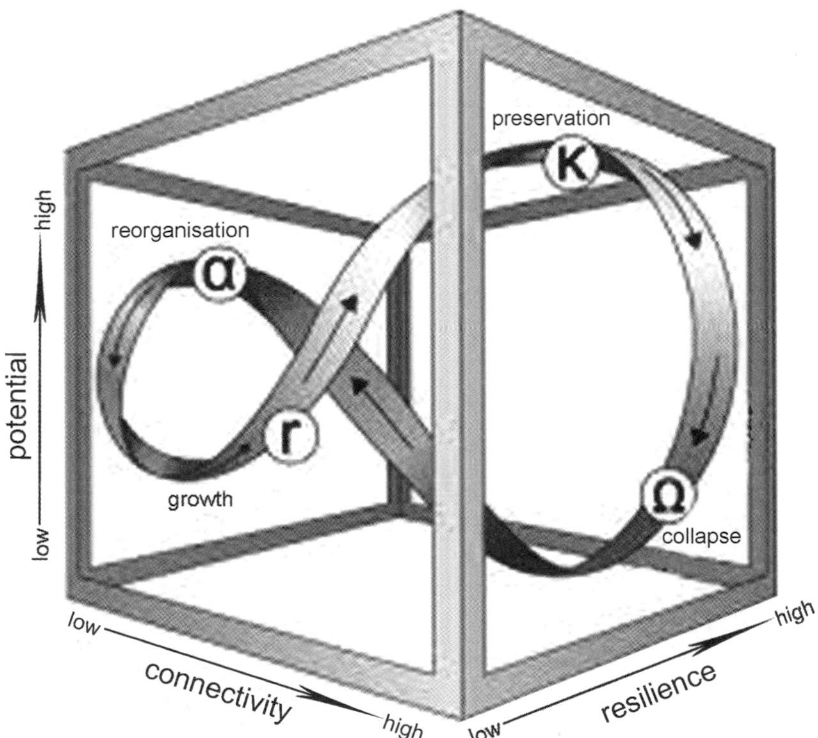

Figure 10.1 Adaptive cycles

Source: From Panarchy *by Lance H. Gunderson and C.S. Holling, eds. Copyright © 2002 Island Press. Reproduced by permission of Island Press, Washington, D.C.*

Resilience is Dynamic

Resilience is a third dimension to the adaptive cycle (Figure 10.1). Resilience of a system is not constant; it expands and contracts within the cycle, interacting with changes in potential and connectedness. Resilience is high during reorganisation and growth, but the system becomes increasingly brittle as connectedness and associated complexity increase. For any given system, resilience is at its lowest at the point where the system fails or collapses, as the perturbation or threat has been of sufficient magnitude to overcome that system's unique ability to absorb the change.

It is important to think of resilience as a changing phenomenon, rather than as a static property for any given system. Improving system resilience is therefore an ongoing process of responding, monitoring, learning, and anticipating, rather than a single activity or intervention (Hollnagel, 2009b; Hollnagel et al., 2010).

In this book resilience is defined in terms of function as 'the intrinsic ability of a system to adjust its functioning prior to, during, or following changes and disturbances, so that it can sustain required operations under both expected and unexpected conditions' (Hollnagel, 2011b). This definition is similar to ecological resilience, defined by Holling as 'the magnitude of disturbance that can be absorbed before the system changes its structure by changing the variables and processes that control behavior' (Holling, 1996: 33). Current understanding of system resilience involves minimising the loss and maximising the recovery (or even surpassing the previous level) of a function, rather than the strictly engineering view of resilience as an elastic property of a system that allows the prevailing structure or processes to continue in their present incarnation. Therefore, resilience is characterised by persistence, adaptability, variability and unpredictability. The nature of change is episodic and results from an interaction between fast and slow processes. Fast and slow processes create both stabilising and regulatory forces, and also destabilising forces, such as opportunity, diversity and resilience.

Similar to socio-ecological systems, socio-technical systems such as health care consist of multiple interacting systems and sub-systems. In terms of the adaptive cycle, these systems are changing and adapting at different rates and attaining different levels of potential, connectedness and resilience. These asynchronous processes can result in an increased complexity and less predictable outcomes. An example in health care is the interaction between innovation in patient care and culture. Changes in the modalities of treatment of illness and injury operate on a fast cycle, with new technology driving innovation in surgical equipment and techniques and the expanding field of genetics resulting in improved pharmaceuticals to treat disease. Culture changes slowly for the most part, however (Braithwaite, Hyde and Pope, 2010), resulting in variable uptake and acceptance of these new drugs and procedures (even where ample evidence exists to support their efficacy).

The theory of systems adapting in cycles, occurring at multiple space and time scales, and driving fast and slow transitions, is known as 'panarchy' (Gunderson and Holling, 2002, Walker et al., 2004). Larger cycles of system change and adaptation will usually constrain smaller cycles; however, cross-scale interactions can result in unpredictable and chaotic events, and failures in one cycle can cascade through the nested cycles, creating a path of destruction. The result is not always negative, but it is likely to be unforeseen, as the following example shows. In 2005, a 16-year-old Australian girl suffered a golfing accident and died in a large public hospital following poor medical management of her condition (Milovanovich, 2008). A large 'disturbance' was applied to the state health care system and the state government in the form of widespread press reporting and consequent community outrage. This resulted in a Special Commission of Inquiry (Garling, 2008), followed by multiple changes to the health care system at multiple levels (Skinner et al., 2009, Stewart and Dwyer, 2010). An example of one of the changes – although the effect of this program is yet to be evaluated – was the introduction of statewide training for all nurses and junior doctors in the detection and management of a deteriorating patient. Reverberations continued in 2011 when, following a state election, the incoming government implemented major structural changes to the state health care system (Foley, 2011).

Larger cycles normally evolve slowly – the growth phase sometimes takes years, or even decades. In health care, success or failure of an intervention is often judged too quickly to allow for changes to occur. One of the *de facto* tools for evaluating team training, for example, is an attitude survey. Attitudes are a component of culture – a slowly cycling system – yet they are frequently measured immediately, following completion of the training (Salas et al., 2006).

In addition to acute perturbations, health care is characterised by predictable, but long-term, changes due to internal or external factors. Throughout the world, population increases will impact on the cost of health care, and, ironically, improvements in the efficacy of health care delivery result in an increased percentage of elderly patients that puts further pressure on resources.

Restructuring, Adaptive Processes and Resilience

As systems thinkers, it is important to view the health care system through multiple lenses when exploring adaptive processes. In terms of physical structure, health care systems have been changing over the last two decades, and we are seeing an increased decentralisation (Braithwaite, Vining and Lazarus 1994). This is partially influenced by technology: as communication systems improve, there is less need for elements of the system to be co-located. So we can have remote biomedical services such as radiology, pathology, and so on, and with the advent of telemedicine, even a remote patient. Although this distributed system provides greater protection and resilience to single point physical perturbations – such as extreme weather events – the increased complexity of the system introduces new paths to failure. Communication may be difficult, for example, when there is no longer frequent personal contact between clinicians and service providers such as imaging. The situation is more complex in some countries – the USA, for example – where decentralisation of physical structures is combined with organisational centralisation, as smaller practices are being acquired by large health systems.

In terms of management structure, new leadership invariably heralds changes to organisational charts, management roles and inter-professional relationships. Research has shown that restructuring does not improve hospital efficiency or effectiveness, with organisations often taking up to three years after the restructure to recover performance to the level achieved prior to the change (Braithwaite, Westbrook and Iedema, 2005). Health care systems that have greater susceptibility to government influence often undergo reorganisation whenever there is a change in political leadership. The NHS, for example, has been in a 'constant state of reform since its inception' (Braithwaite, Westbrook and Iedema, 2005). If the trade-off between exploiting the current structure and exploring ideas for new structures veers too far in the direction of exploration, the system can end up in a state of 'eternal boiling' (Axelrod and Cohen, 2000: 43) or constant disarray. In health care, in addition to government policy and decisions, there are also large influencers in the form of corporations such as technological and pharmaceutical companies. While governments tend to sponsor top-down influence, technology and pharmaceutical companies can disturb the system at multiple levels, from political donations down to approaches appealing to individual doctors, or advertising targeted at patients.

Targeted interventions, such as team and inter-professional training, and introduction of technology have made small inroads into improving safety, but system-wide improvements have not been realised. Production can be improved in the short term by introducing mechanisms to reduce system variability. However, longer term, reduced variability results in reduced resilience. So, while the system may appear to be performing efficiently and effectively, over time it is susceptible to smaller disturbances and adverse events are more likely to occur. Constraining the adaptive cycle often requires expensive patches to fix arising problems, and this contributes to an increasingly brittle system. Fixes – like barriers – are Safety-I thinking solutions that increase complexity, and ultimately risk increasing the number of paths to failure (Braithwaite, 2006). As Axelrod and Cohen caution: 'Do not sow large failures when reaping small efficiencies' (Axelrod and Cohen, 2000). Meadows talks about system leverage points, or the most effective places to intervene in a system to trigger change (Meadows, 1999). Leverage points – and the direction to apply leverage – are frequently counter-intuitive; modifying the information and control components of a system is usually more effective than changing the physical or structural arrangement of the organisation.

While recent structural (Braithwaite, 2006) and training innovations (Salas et al., 2008) have been implemented from the view of health care as a function of patient care, some health care professionals may view the same system along professional lines. The disconnect between management-imposed structure and workplace culture can contribute to differences in work as envisioned by management and work as it is actually done in hospital wards and operating theatres (Braithwaite and Westbrook, 2005; Dekker, 2011a). This difference may be reflected in the prevalence of violations of documented workplace procedures. Aligning management and clinical approaches may prove fruitful; Woods talks about this as real time resilience being generated through both a bottom-up and top-down process (Woods, 2006). Aligning the various modes of change may allow system-level processes to be simplified. So, for example, if structural change, inter-professional training, introduction of new technology, and physical relocation of facilities and resources can be achieved under a common purpose, system complexity may be reduced.

To understand – and ultimately improve – system resilience, we need to be able to view the big picture, the macro outcomes in addition to the micro. To do that, the patient-centred view of the clinician needs to be considered in combination with the service-provider view of the manager. We need to accept the dualistic and nested nature of health care as a process of autonomous action within a bureaucratic system. We need to provide a 'safe space' for autonomy. This is not inconsistent with safe system operation: we consider a desktop computer, for example, as a relatively predictable and effective machine. Yet at the level of the tiny analogue transistor, millions of which make up the integrated circuitry that forms the computer, we observe non-linear behaviour. And at the level of the electrons that flow through the transistor, behaviour can be chaotic and unpredictable. In a similar manner, it may be possible in large health care systems to have a degree of autonomy at the interface with the patient, yet predictability and effectiveness at the level of the organisation.

Conclusion

We should not be in such a hurry to 'change the system', either by restructuring or by insisting on micro-reforms by top-down means. But it is difficult to show restraint, because health care professionals and managers are trained to look at what is wrong, and to try and fix it. However, the effects of a restructure can result in a loss of function followed by a period of recovery with sub-par performance that is not dissimilar to the effect of an extreme weather event. There is an old heuristic in aviation that when you encounter an 'emergency', the first thing you must do is 'sit on your hands'. Do we need to sit on our hands in health care, and improve our learning and understanding of the system before rushing to implement change? It would seem so. We need to establish what is working well now, rather than immediately imposing what we imagine we would like to have in the future. We need to examine overall patterns, over longer time frames, rather than try for quick fixes. Knowing that every change has the potential to add complexity to the system, perhaps we need to consider a synoptic incremental (Camillus, 1982) approach: when dealing with a complex adaptive system, the way forward should be evolution, not revolution.

Chapter 11
Relying on Resilience: Too Much of a Good Thing?

Robert L. Wears and Charles A. Vincent

Introduction

At first glance, this chapter's subject may seem out of place; resilience is generally thought of as an unalloyed good, something that care delivery organisations should always want more of. However, no silver lining is without its cloud, and there is reason to believe that in some circumstances health care organisations and their work systems might rely too heavily on resilience to promote safe and effective performance; in others, they might misuse resilience to resist a needed change. This chapter explores the negative potential of resilience – its overuse and misuse – and suggests some possible causes for this problem.

Too Much Resilience?

Can an organisation be too resilient? It is hard to conceive of one having too great an ability to adapt to sustain its key operations. But, there may be many ways in which adaptation might be enacted, many ways in which key operations might be sustained, and in addition, many views on what might constitute key operations. Thus, a reasonable question might be the appropriate degree to which an organisation relies on resilience to achieve this goal (as opposed to other possible means [Vincent et al., 2010]). An important corollary question is to ask whose resilience is employed in this effort and whether problems in one part of the organisation, or externally, are requiring a resilient response in another part.

While it might therefore be difficult to conceive of an organisation being too resilient, there may be ways in which resilience is deployed inappropriately, wastefully or even dangerously. Firstly, an organisation might, for instance, depend on resilience too much to achieve routine success, frittering away a valuable adaptive resource on the everyday that might better be husbanded for greater or less tractable threats. Secondly, it might spend too much of its time and effort in adapting to issues that might not have been real challenges, and thus degrade its own ability to sustain key operations in a sort of disorderly, continuous boiling (Axelrod and Cohen, 2000). Thirdly, it might employ resilience unevenly across organisational levels and create a sort of co-dependency. Here, front-line resilience leads to short-term 'fixes' that put off more fundamental, long-term solutions; or, it allows upper management to protect itself from inconvenient truths and shift accountability for failures to front-line workers. And finally, an organisation might use resilience in support of mistaken or erroneous goals – for example, resiliently resisting a needed change. Any or all of these scenarios might co-exist and reinforce an unhealthy dependency on resilience.

Case Studies

To illustrate these possibilities in health care, we present two scenarios in which we propose that resilience is deployed inappropriately. In the first, a regular but short-term crisis in the supply of a drug is resolved by imposing a solution which requires an unusual, and generally unnecessary, degree of watchfulness and adaptation on the part of front-line staff. In the second, we reflect more widely on how problems of basic reliability are routinely overcome by resilient adaptations and workarounds which, while successful in the short term, may have very damaging longer term consequences.

Compensating for Shortages: Imposing Resilience on the Front Line

Drug shortages have become endemic in Western health care systems over the past quarter century (Institute for Safe Medication Practices, 2010). Propofol, an important drug commonly used in

US emergency departments (EDs), has been in critically short supply for several years (Jensen and Rappaport, 2010). Propofol is widely used for procedural sedation because of its favourable safety profile and its rapidity of action: the onset of sedation occurs within 40–60 seconds after intravenous injection, and its effect wears off in three to five minutes. These properties (and others) make it a first-choice drug for brief procedures (such as fracture reduction) in the ED. While alternatives are available, none has the combination of speed and safety offered by propofol, and practitioners are less comfortable with them due to a lower frequency of use. Thus, hospitals routinely struggle to obtain adequate supplies of propofol.

The hospital in this example was able to locate a supply of propofol pre-packaged in syringes, rather than in vials, from which it must be drawn up into syringes, as is typical. Propofol is one of only a few injectable drugs that have a characteristic appearance; it is milky white (most other injectables are clear). But, another injectable commonly used in the ED – the antibiotic benzathine penicillin – is similarly milky white, and also comes in pre-packaged syringes (see Figure 11.1). But there is an important difference between the two drugs beyond the differences in their indications and mechanisms of action; they require mutually exclusive routes of injection. Benzathine penicillin is only used intramuscularly (IM), while propofol is only used intravenously (IV). IM injection of propofol is ineffective and can be associated with tissue necrosis at the injection site; but worse, IV injection of benzathine penicillin has been fatal (Smetzer and Cohen, 1998).

Managers understood the potential for confusion between the two preparations, but went ahead because most clinical areas in the hospital commonly use only one of these drugs (the ED was the main exception, where both are commonly used). They added a label to the propofol syringes, sent an email to staff warning about the change, and trusted that the staff would be able to work it out. Other potential solutions (for example, transferring propofol from syringes into sterile bottles) were rejected as too costly and risking bacterial contamination. On this basis, the organisation stocked the new formulation of propofol, meeting important organisational goals but necessarily introducing a potential risk, on the assumption that 'the staff can sort it out.'

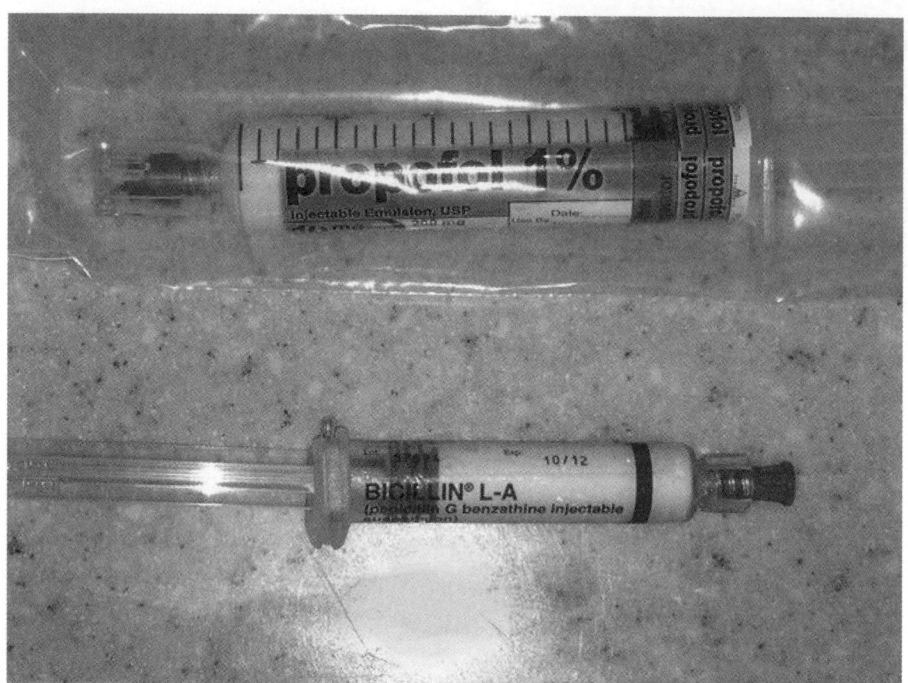

Figure 11.1 Propofol (upper) and benzathine penicillin (lower) have similar appearances and packaging

To be sure, the reasoning behind this decision did not explicitly include resilience, but rather was based on appeals for greater care and vigilance by the ED staff, so the dependence on resilience here is implicit, not explicit – but it is nonetheless present. This example also illustrates the cross-level complexities of resilience and the potential to fail by working at cross purposes (Woods and Branlat, 2011a). In this case, the organisation solved an overall problem by increasing the demand for resilient adaptation on one group of workers in an acute-chronic trade-off: the short-term problem of a present drug shortage was resolved by risking the long-term problem of a fatal misadministration in the future (Hoffman and Woods, 2011: Woods and Branlat, 2011b). The ability to depend on the resilience of the ED staff (to deal with the 'surprise' of the look-alike packaging) allowed the organisation to choose a riskier option than it otherwise might have.

Resilience as Compensation for Poor Reliability

Reliability is commonly defined as 'the probability of a component, or system, functioning correctly over a given period of time under a given set of operating conditions' (Storey, 1996). In this context, 'functioning correctly' refers to functioning according to some given specification. Reliability is usually expressed in terms of failure rate per hour for systems operating continuously, or probability of failure on demand for demand-based systems. For example, electronic and software systems possess clear specifications and the reliability of these systems is assessed against this specification in terms of defined inputs and outputs.

In health care systems, or indeed in other complex systems, it can be more difficult to define with precision just what 'functioning correctly' means. The most important reason for this is that the reliability can only be strictly assessed against a precisely defined process, and many health care problems and processes have an irreducible variability. While much of this variation and adaptation is appropriate and necessary, given a heterogeneous, variable, ambiguous problem space (Ashby, 1958), it cannot be denied that much flexibility in health care stems not from necessary adaptation, but from a casualness that leads to a dependence on resilience as a means of compensating for poor reliability.

For example, Burnett and colleagues studied four clinical sub-systems in seven hospitals in the British NHS: clinical information in surgical outpatient clinics, prescribing for hospital inpatients, equipment in theatres, and insertion of peripheral intravenous lines. They examined the reliability of these sub-systems and the factors involved where failures occurred (Burnett et al., 2012). Reliability was defined as a 100 per cent fault free operation (for example, if all patients had all the required information available at the time of their appointment). Reliability was found to be between 81 per cent and 87 per cent for the sub-systems studied, with significant variation between organisations. Put another way, the clinical sub-systems studied failed on 13–19 per cent of occasions. About 20 per cent of reliability failures were associated with a potential risk of harm. These levels of reliability strongly suggest the underlying processes, roles, and responsibilities are inadequate for the tasks they serve. If such levels of reliability were typical, it would mean doctors must deal with missing clinical information for three in every 20 outpatients seen; missing or faulty equipment in one of seven operations performed; and that nurses and pharmacists must waste time correcting problems and searching for records or equipment for four or five patients every day on a typical 30-bed ward. On this basis it is hardly surprising that patient safety is routinely compromised in NHS hospitals, or that clinical staff come to accept poor reliability as part of everyday life and exalt resilience as a means of compensating for it.

Responding Resiliently: Workarounds and Adaptations

When asked how they dealt with instances of poor reliability, staff described the workarounds they had developed; for example, obtaining information from patients rather than their health records, or using disposable gloves as tourniquets. Risks could not be assessed directly for many workarounds, but in some cases, risks were taken, such as making clinical decisions without information, or transferring used sharps to sharps bins in remote locations. These workarounds are an example of 'first order problem solving' – adapting one's work to cope with the basic inefficiencies of the system. Clinical staff are extremely adept at this but their facility in compensation can inhibit more fundamental system change. Clinicians display resilient behaviour in adapting to and recovering from potentially dangerous situations, but for the most part, resilience was only required because reliability was poor.

While workarounds are often both ubiquitous and necessary, since formal procedures are always underspecified, they can lead to a progressive disconnect between work-as-imagined by managers and work-as-performed on the front line. This gap effectively prevents organisational learning; as front-line workers become better and better at finding ways to meet their goals (Wears and Cook, 2010; Woods and Hollnagel, 2006), the problems they surmount disappear from both their own and their managers' views (Tucker, 2010; Tucker and Edmondson, 2002; Tucker and Edmondson, 2003).

In addition, by (in effect) training workers to expect that things typically do not work (by asking them routinely to fit square pegs into round holes), organisations remove the potential for engineered interlocks to work as designed. Health care workers are so used to adapting to surprises – such as drugs coming in different packaging this week, or devices or connectors not fitting together – that they have been conditioned to ignore the warning signals that they have picked up the wrong drug, or that two devices ought not be connected.

These two factors create a type of co-dependency problem, where well-intended attempts to resolve immediate issues allow underlying problems to continue, and in fact create resistance towards more fundamental solutions.

Burnout and Failure to Learn: The Costs of Relying on Resilience

Excessive reliance on resilience is expensive in the long run in a number of ways. Firstly, as previously noted, the capacity to respond, monitor, learn, and anticipate is finite. While using it commonly and frequently can help develop and maintain the ability to adapt, excessive use of the ordinary can leave it depleted when faced with the extraordinary. Secondly, it can lead to frustration, cynicism, burnout, and turnover among front-line workers, who become exhausted by the task of swimming upstream against an unending tide of small, annoying problems (Tucker and Edmondson, 2003).

Relying unnecessarily on the resilience and adaptability of clinical staff also has profound consequences for the wider organisation. When staff go to find missing equipment or they adapt procedures because of lack of clinical information, they are generally performing an important service for the particular patient they are caring for. This first-order problem solving is effective in the short term, but prevents problems from surfacing as learning opportunities. Ongoing problems of poor reliability become invisible precisely because front-line staff adapt and either fail to complain or, worse, come to feel that there is no point in complaining. While first-order problem solving is admirable, it needs to be followed by second-order problem solving; this involves patching the immediate problem, but also letting the relevant people know that the problem has occurred, so that preventative – rather than merely compensatory – action can follow.

Resilience can, therefore, act against an organisation's longer-term interests by burying problems that are thus never resolved and remain a threat to patients. Counter-intuitively, positive personal and organisational attributes can prevent organisational change in the following way:

- First, individual vigilance, resourcefulness and problem solving ability militate against change, as we have discussed.
- Second, this is compounded and reinforced by a system that makes sure that nurses are constantly used to the full, which means that they only have time to care for patients and not to address – much less resolve – wider organisational issues.
- Third, managers, who actually have the power to resolve these problems in the longer term, are not aware of them and so not engaged to resolve them.

Why is Resilience Over-used or Misused?

Behaviours persist in social systems because someone benefits from them; in this chapter we explore some potential reasons for the misapplication of resilience in health care, in terms of benefits to the organisation and the individual.

Organisation

Care delivery organisations unwittingly adopt resilient solutions to problems they face. This use is unwitting in two senses. Firstly, it is an inadvertent by-product of the way problems are managed, not an explicit choice on the part of those in charge (many of whom would be only superficially familiar with the concept). And secondly, much of resilience and Safety-II thinking clashes with the rhetoric dominant in health care, which glorifies a Taylorist, 'measure and manage' approach characterised by increasingly prescriptive, feed-forward control; for example, 'evidence-based medicine' (Evidence-Based Medicine Working Group, 1992), clinical practice guidelines (Eddy, 1990), or the renewed emphasis on individual accountability (Goldmann, 2006).

Despite its clashing with articulated ways of managing clinical work, care delivery organisations employ resilience because it is serves other useful purposes beyond being a means of simply getting the work done (Cook and Nemeth, 2010, Dekker, Nyce and Myers, 2012). In particular, it allows the more powerful layers of the organisation to avoid uncomfortable problems. As noted above, hospitals cannot learn from their history because in a sense, they have no history; the stories of near failures and how they are routinely overcome are encapsulated in the tight, difficult to penetrate social networks of the front-line workers. The organisation benefits because unknown issues do not pose the problem of potentially expensive, threatening, or disruptive actions. Further, this implicit reliance on resilience allows the organisation to deflect responsibility to the front-line workers when thing eventually do go wrong, preserving the reputation and privileges of the powerful with some 'soporific injunctions about better training' (Perrow, 1986). Finally, the appearance that ordinary operations seem to come off safely and as planned reinforces a comforting, rationalist illusion of control; the idea that the organisation's processes and procedures are leading to a better, more controllable, less chaotic and less threatening world (Cook and Nemeth, 2010, Dekker, Nyce and Myers, 2012).

Individual

Front line workers also find beneficial aspects to an over-reliance on resilience. First, resilience offers a better fit with the long-standing, guild-oriented models of professionalism held by clinicians. The well-documented resistance to 'foreign' interventions such as Lean, practice guidelines, standardisation, evidence-based medicine, etc., 'exemplifies the tenaciousness of this form of expression of professional identity' (McDonald et al.; 2006, Radnor, Holweg and Waring, 2012; Timmermans and Berg, 2003).

In addition, resilience fits well with the 'heroic narrative' widely shared among health professionals, particularly doctors (Dekker, 2011b). By substituting the irrational or recalcitrant 'system' in place of illness or injury as the 'villain' to be overcome in this narrative, health professionals maintain their central role as *the* important actors in achieving success, thus ensuring their special status and privileges in society.

Conclusion

Despite the dominance of Safety-I thinking in health care and abundant rhetoric favouring more centralised, prescriptive, 'rational' control of care processes, health care organisations paradoxically and unknowingly use resilient strategies to address some of their problems. When overused or misused, these strategies lead to additional problems for care delivery organisations, in terms of workarounds leading to reduced safety and organisational learning; increased staff effort, cynicism, frustration and burnout; and resistance to needed change. This misapplication occurs and persists because it provides useful benefits to both care delivery organisations and individual practitioners.

Chapter 12
Mindful Organising and Resilient Health Care

Kathleen M. Sutcliffe and Karl E. Weick

Introduction

In a June 2012 commencement address delivered to graduating students at Williams College in Williamstown, Massachusetts in the USA, American physician and journalist Atul Gawande described the criticality of resilient health care and ways to achieve it (Gawande, 2012). Using surgery as an example, he acknowledged that although surgery has become relatively safe and routine, health care institutions continue to vary widely in their outcomes, especially with mortality rates.

Gawande observed that the foremost question is what accounts for these differences? It is reasonable to think (as he had for quite some time) that the best institutions are simply better at preventing things from going wrong. Gawande went on to say he was surprised that recent findings by researchers at the University of Michigan contradicted this logic. The findings he referred to were reported in a study of hospital mortality associated with inpatient surgery. Amir Ghaferi and colleagues at Michigan's Surgical Collaborative for Outcomes Research and Evaluation (see Ghaferi, Birkmeyer and Dimick, 2009a, 2009b) discovered that low mortality hospitals do not do a better job of controlling risks or preventing post-surgical complications. High and low mortality hospitals experienced relatively similar complication rates after surgeries. What differed was the rate at which the high mortality hospitals 'failed to rescue'. Low-mortality hospitals were more proficient at recognising and managing serious complications as they unfolded.

We interpret proficient recognising and managing of complications as an instance of *mindful organising*. Our interest is not in 'failure to rescue' as a static metric. Instead, we are interested in the processes implied in *rescuing, recognising* and *managing* emerging complications before they turn into a fatal flaw. To gain insight into how failures to rescue are reduced, our referent is *failing* to rescue, or – more specifically – its obverse, *rescuing*. Rescuing is treated as an instance of the more general pattern wherein organising that leads to failing or succeeding is dependent on the extent to which that organising is mindful. Mindful organising is specified as five complementary processes that improve ongoing attention and intervention. Those five processes involve preoccupation with failure, avoidance of simplifying interpretations, sensitivity to operations, commitments to resilience (i.e. capacity building), and flexible decision structures that defer to expertise.

Our analysis presumes that resilience is something a system does, not something a system has. As systems organise more or less mindfully, their ongoing actions are more or less likely to accommodate and adjust to complicating surprise. We propose that capabilities to act resiliently are enabled and enacted through processes of mindful organising. Thus, mechanisms of mindful organising underpin resilient health care. We elaborate this perspective by brief discussion of organising processes implicit in rescuing, followed by a more detailed discussion of mindful organising itself.

Rescuing

Rescuing, whether successful or unsuccessful, involves 'recursive interactions between interpreting and updating' in a dynamic, unfolding situation (Rudolph, Morrison and Carroll, 2009: 740). As sociologist Marianne Paget (1988) observed, health care work is a process of discovery – it is discovered in the actions of apprehending, inferring, testing, experimenting, tracking and following courses of events as they unfold. Rescuing involves discovery under pressure, pressure from a deteriorating patient and pressure on the relations among members of the treatment team itself. Lagadec (1993) has portrayed increased pressure as a brutal audit that exposes weakness in relations among team members. These weaknesses may arise in the way people interrelate their task performances (e.g., Weick and Roberts, 1993) as well as in their expectations of one another around issues of trust, trustworthiness, and self-respect (Campbell, 1990). Consequently, it is both more useful and accurate to think about resilient heath care as a dynamic ongoing accomplishment.

Cook and Woods (1994: 273) set the stage for the fundamentals of rescuing: 'Nothing can be discovered in the world without attention; no intended change in the world can be effected without shifting attention to the thing being acted upon.' What makes it more difficult to recognise and manage post-operative complications is that the system is trying to deal with a continuously evolving situation by imposing discrete, discontinuous concepts and diagnoses. Discrete concepts imposed on ongoing perceptions typically lag behind what is observed to have just occurred. Discrete categories are usually imposed a little too late and, because of their discreteness, miss some of the continuing change. Events are always a little farther along and a little different from how we imagine (Weick, 2011). The size of the gap created by this disjunction is dependent on such things as the frequency of updating, the extent to which the leading diagnosis is free of fixation and confirmation bias, the composition of the unit and quality of interactions, and the extent to which the unit is organised to redirect its attention and performance while members continue to maintain trust, trustworthiness, and self-respect. To reduce the size of this gap in the face of adversity and to continue to perform well is the essence of resilient acting (Sutcliffe and Vogus, 2003). But concepts too play a significant role in determining the size of this gap. As William James put it, 'The intellectual life of man consists almost wholly in his substitution of a conceptual order for the perceptual order in which his experience originally comes' (James, 1996: 50–51). James's summary is stated at an individual level of analysis. Multi-person systems potentially should be better at recognising and managing complications because their collective conceptual substitutions are broader, more diverse, collectively more comprehensive, and better suited to rescuing. But that possibility depends on how the system is organised.

As the organising becomes more mindful, the likelihood of rescuing becomes more likely.

Rescuing itself occurs as people 'amass and integrate uncertain, incomplete, and changing evidence ... (P)ractitioners make provisional assessments based on partial and uncertain data. These assessments are incrementally updated and revised as more evidence comes in' (Cook and Woods, 1994: 274–5). Rudolph, Morrison and Carroll (2009: 748) develop a similar evolving picture of rescuing in their model of action-based inquiry. For them, activities such as rescuing involve at least three properties: (1) information cues that become available only by taking action; (2) a deteriorating situation with its attendant pressure to act on the leading diagnosis or to cultivate a new one; and (3) changes in the characteristics of the environment and the stream of cues that become available as a result of action. In both of the above descriptions it is clear that rescuing consists of ongoing, dynamic practices. Borrowing from Langley and Tsoukas (2012: 13), rescuing involves the 'reconstitution of an evolving present.'

Mindful Organising

To move from the specifics of a process view of 'failure to rescue' to a more general framework that deals with organising to rescue – to manage surprises as they unfold – we dwell briefly on organising to establish some boundaries. Organising is about assembling interdependent actions into sensible sequences that generate sensible outcomes (Weick, 1979: 3). In other words, 'Organizing is a constant sensemaking process, a constant effort to impose order on our perceptions, experiences, and expectations' (Gabriel, 2008: 212). Organisation, therefore, is an emergent outcome of processes that accomplish ongoing mutual adjustment. This mutual adjusting, as noted earlier, is visible in activities such as joint interpreting, discovering, testing, and redefining. The goal is an improved grasp of what in fact may be evolving.

Collectively, processes of mindful organising assist people to focus attention on perceptual details that are typically lost when they coordinate their actions and share their interpretations and conceptions (Baron and Misovich, 1999). Mindful organising reduces the loss of detail by increasing the quality of attention across the organisation, enhancing people's alertness and awareness so that they can detect discrepancies and subtle ways in which situations and contexts vary and call for contingent responding (Weick and Sutcliffe, 2006, 2007). Mindfulness generates enhanced awareness of context, which then makes situations more meaningful. That increase in meaningfulness occurs because there is more information about failures, simplifications, capacities, and expertise associated with present and emerging challenges (Weick and Sutcliffe, 2007). Without these contextual inputs, awareness is more likely to be simplified into familiar categories that have been applied in the past. There is nothing wrong with influence from the past, but it tends to be stripped of context and subject to the editing of hindsight.

Processes of Mindful Organising

Mindful organising is a function of a collective's (such as a sub-unit or work group) attention to context and capacities to act. It provides a basis for people to interact as they develop, refine and update shared understandings of the situations they face and their capabilities to act on those understandings. When work-group members focus sustained attention on operations (e.g., how their work is unfolding presently) they enhance the likelihood that they will develop, deepen, and update a shared understanding of their local work context and emerging vulnerabilities. As they understand better what they face, they enhance the collective's ability to marshal the necessary resources and capabilities to act on that understanding in a flexible manner that is tailored to the unexpected contingency.

Mindful organising is *enabled* when leaders and organisational members pay close attention to shaping the social and relational infrastructure of the organisation (Weick and Roberts, 1993; Weick, 2011). And it is *enacted* through five interrelated processes and associated practices (Weick, Sutcliffe and Obstfeld, 1999; Vogus and Sutcliffe, 2007a, 2007b). Together these strengthen the system's (e.g., team, unit, organisation) overall safety infrastructure (e.g., culture) and capabilities to act resiliently. We describe the enabling and enacting of mindful organising below.

Enabling Mindful Organising

When organisational members face situations where their private view is at odds with a majority view, they often feel threatened. Feelings of threat reduce their willingness to speak up about potential problems (Blatt et al., 2006). These dynamics may be particularly acute in health care settings where work is hierarchical, heterarchical (see Chapter 6), and distributed, where patients' conditions evolve and change over time, where transitions and handoffs between providers are frequent, where team memberships change, and where professionals differ in power, social status, professional languages, and ways of communicating. To counteract these tendencies and to encourage people to speak up and question interpretations, it is necessary to establish a context of trust and respect. In contexts where respect is the norm, people are both more likely to communicate their interpretations to others and also are more likely through this communication to generate a shared interpretation (Christianson and Sutcliffe, 2009). These results lessen the likelihood of misperceptions, misconceptions, and misunderstandings (Schulman, 2004).

In addition to building a social-relational context of respect and trust, attention must be paid to the interrelating of activities (Weick, 2011). Studies show that when the crews of aircraft carriers are more aware of how their contributions interrelate with those of others, they tend to have fewer serious accidents and errors (Weick and Roberts, 1993). Heedful interrelating is a pattern of differentiation and integration through which individual action contributes to a larger pattern of shared action and in which individuals understand how their actions fit into the larger action (Weick and Roberts, 1993). When people interrelate heedfully, they first understand how a system is configured to achieve some goal and they see their work as a contribution to the system and not as a standalone activity. Second, they visualise the meshing of their job with other people's jobs to accomplish the goals of the system. And third, they maintain a conscious awareness of both configurations and contributions as they perform their duties.

Respectful interaction and heedful interrelating generate shared interpretation and shared action and form the social-relational foundation for mindful organising, and ultimately for acting resiliently. When trust and respect are absent, providers often silence themselves either because they think speaking up won't make a difference or that speaking up might harm their image or relationship with their supervisor (Blatt et al., 2006; Edmondson, 2003). Vogus (2004) studied 125 nursing units in 13 hospitals and found that higher levels of respectful interacting and heedful interrelating were associated with lower levels of medication errors and patient falls.

Enacting Mindful Organising

A social–relational infrastructure built around trust and contributions is necessary for mindful organising but not sufficient. That infrastructure must be organised and enacted through conduct that enables organisational members to recognise emerging problems earlier and to manage them more decisively. Thus, rescuing should vary as a function of the extent to which organisations and their sub-units establish processes and practices aimed at (a) a preoccupation with failure to better understand the health of the overall system; (b) avoiding simplifying assumptions and interpretations about the world; (c) a sensitivity to current operations and their effects; (d) a commitment to developing resilience; and (e) creating flexible decision structures so that decisions can migrate to experts.

1. *Preoccupation with failure.* A preoccupation with failure reflects an ongoing wariness that analytic error is embedded in ongoing activities (Weick, Sutcliffe and Obstfeld, 1999: 91). This wariness (Reason, 1997) drives proactive and pre-emptive analyses of possible vulnerabilities such as normalising, crude labels, inattention to current operations, rigid adherence to routines, and inflexible hierarchies. Preoccupation also treats small failures, mistakes, and near misses as indicators of potentially larger problems. Worrying about failure is a distinctive quality of mindful organising. People pay close attention to what needs to go right, what could go wrong, how it could go wrong, and what has gone wrong. This does not mean that people are paralysed by worries about making mistakes or thinking about how to fix

or prevent the last problem; rather, it means that people actively search for seemingly insignificant anomalies that might not warrant attention but might indicate that the system is acting in unexpected ways. Preoccupation with failure is an effort to avoid hubris, the liabilities of success (Miller, 1993), and the arrogance of optimism (Landau and Chisholm, 1995), all of which contribute to inertia and mindlessness.

Preoccupation with failure may seem antithetical to the spirit of Safety-II. But not so if we consider safety as a dynamic 'non-event' (Weick, 1987). Safety is a non-event because successful outcomes rarely call attention to themselves. In other words, because safe outcomes are constant, there is nothing to pay attention to. This can decrease vigilance, the sense of vulnerability, and the quality of attention while it also increases the propensity toward complacency and inertia, across the organisation. All can be deadly. Ongoing wariness has a better track record. 'Ongoing' implies continuing with whatever is working or succeeding. 'Wariness' means awareness of traps in those efforts to keep going. Moreover, ongoing wariness is critical to counteract tendencies toward confirmation bias and positive asymmetry. Positive asymmetry (Cerulo, 2006) is the tendency to focus on and exaggerate the best-case characteristics or the most optimistic outlook or outcomes – often until it is too late.

2. *Avoiding simplified interpretations.* Organisations or units that avoid simplifying interpretations do not take the past as an infallible guide to the future. Instead, they socialise their members to make fewer assumptions, to actively question received wisdom, to uncover blind spots and bring more perspectives to bear on problems and decisions so that key variables are not overlooked. Simplifications are troublesome because they give people a false sense that they know precisely what they face. They also limit the precautions people take and the number of undesired consequences they imagine. In part this is an issue of requisite variety. The law of requisite variety asserts that the variety of a system such as an organisation, team, or individual, must be as great as the variety of the environment that it is trying to regulate (Ashby, 1956). It is often assumed that variety in any form is 'requisite', but, in fact, the type of variety that is brought to bear

is critical (see Dimov, Shepherd and Sutcliffe, 2007). The variety sought by more mindful organisations is that which provides insight into their particular environments and ongoing activities. In other words, through questioning assumptions and offering diverse alternatives, a reluctance to simplify interpretations enlarges the interpretive variety of a work group such that they are able to see more possibilities. Consequently, reluctance to simplify interpretations is the means by which organisations can create and draw on requisite variety, and more effectively make adjustments to unfolding situations.

3. *Sensitivity to current operations.* Sensitivity to operations means creating and maintaining an integrated big picture of current situations through ongoing attention to real-time information. Organisations that have real-time information and situational understanding can forestall the compounding of small problems or failures by making a number of small adjustments. Small adjustments are opportunities to stop mistakes and errors from lining up in such a way that they combine into a bigger crisis. Many untoward events originate in latent failures; loopholes in the system's defences such as defects in supervision, training, briefings or hazard identification (Reason, 1997). Being in close touch with what is happening here and now means that the downstream effects of these latent problems can be reduced or in some way compensated for.

4. *Commitment to resilience.* People – individually or collectively – try to anticipate possible dangers by creating, improving and revising plans and procedures to incorporate the lessons from past experience. This is consistent with Hollnagel's observations about Safety-I (see Chapter 1). But it is impossible to eliminate uncertainty or create procedures to anticipate all situations and conditions that shape people's work (Wildavsky, 1988). Thus committed organisations continually enlarge individual and organisational capabilities. The larger the repertoire of actions a system can take, the more problems it can afford to see. If you have no way of managing the problems in front of you, then you are less likely to recognise them to begin with (Westrum, 1994).

5. *Creating flexible decision structures*. Flexible decision structures (also referred to as deference to expertise) (Weick, Sutcliffe and Obstfeld, 1999; Weick and Sutcliffe, 2007) arise when, in the face of problems or unexpected events, a collective pools the necessary expertise and utilises it by enabling the person or people with the greater expertise in handling the problem at hand to make decisions, regardless of formal rank. Typically in hierarchical organisations, important choices are made by important decision makers who can participate in many choices. Mindful organising privileges a different priority. When unexpected problems arise, the organisation loosens the designation of who is the 'important' decision maker in order to allow decision making to migrate along with problems (see Roberts, Stout and Halpern, 1994: 622). The result is that hierarchical rank is subordinated to expertise, which increases the likelihood that new capabilities will be matched with new problems, assuring that emerging problems will get quick attention before they blow up. In other words, the organisation has more skills and expertise to draw on. This flexibility enables the system to deal with inevitable uncertainty and imperfect knowledge (Weick, Sutcliffe and Obstfeld, 1999).

Mindful organising, with its emphasis on improving system awareness and alertness, as well as capacities to act, is an important means to rescuing and resilience. Although specific organising practices naturally vary from context to context, collectivities that organise for mindfulness exhibit the following types of behaviours (see Vogus and Sutcliffe, 2007a):

- Unit members prospectively spend time identifying activities they do not want to go wrong, and imagining how they might go wrong.
- Unit members incessantly talk about surprises, mishaps, their prevention, and what can be learned from them.
- In handoffs or reports to oncoming staff, people discuss what to look out for.
- Unit leaders and members actively seek out alternative perspectives and encourage each other to voice concerns and express different opinions.
- People report that there is a context of trust and respect and they feel safe to voice problems and tough issues.

- People interact often enough during the day to build a clear picture of what is happening here and now.
- People have access to a variety of resources whenever unexpected surprises crop up.
- People have a good 'map' of each other's unique talents and skills and pool this expertise when problems arise that they cannot solve.
- People consistently work to improve their competence and develop new response repertoires.

Moreover, research affirms the salutary effects of mindful organising. For example, a qualitative longitudinal study of a paediatric intensive care unit (PICU) showed that the introduction of mindful organising practices was associated with lower levels of patient deterioration – an exceptional achievement given the medical fragility of the patients (Roberts et al., 2005). In another study, Knox, Simpson and Garite (1999) found that hospital obstetrical units distinguished by the features of mindful organising had better safety performance and fewer malpractice claims. Finally, Vogus and Sutcliffe (2007a, 2007b) found an inverse association between mindful organising, unit medication errors and patient falls.

Conclusion

A chapter focused on failures to rescue at first glance may seem to be an example of Safety-I; which, in a book devoted to Safety-II, may seem ironic. But that assessment is incorrect. It shows the shortcomings of the contrast between reactive, past-oriented Safety-I and proactive, future-oriented Safety-II. The shortcomings lie in the neglect of the current, ongoing enactive, which we might call Safety-III. Safety-III – enactive safety – embodies the reactive and proactive and therefore both bridges the past and future and synthesises their lessons and prospects into current action. That is, as we have argued, mindful organising involves both anticipating and rebounding in the face of surprise and complication.

Recognition and management of the unanticipated involves systems in motion. The combination of a preoccupation with failure, reluctance to simplify interpretations, and sensitivity to operations, is enacted to anticipate vulnerabilities, contingencies, or discrepancies in order either to preclude them or to prevent their further complication (Weick and Sutcliffe, 2007). Jointly, these three processes enable a rich representation of the complexity of potential threats. The further enactment of a commitment to resilience and flexible decision structures jointly constructs the pool of expertise and the capacity to use that expertise in a flexible manner that allows for swift recovery. Taken as a whole, these five processes constitute mindful organising. They represent a style of working in which actions such as those involved in rescuing, interpreting, and updating are tied together by ongoing orderly interrelating. This style of joint work is difficult to sustain because it involves complex relationships. But creating, maintaining, and strengthening those relationships is worth the effort because their breakdown constructs one pathway through which preventable hospital mortality gets heightened.

PART III
The Nature and Practice of Resilient Health Care

Chapter 13
Separating Resilience from Success

Rollin J. Fairbanks, Shawna Perry, William Bond and Robert L. Wears

The Association of Resilience with Outcome: Separating Resilience from Success

Outcome is a powerful signal, and we tend to associate resilience with successful outcomes. From this superficial view, a system with a positive outcome seems resilient, while one with a negative outcome does not. However, if resilience engineering is to progress from being a descriptive field to an applied one improving the overall performance of complex socio-technical systems, some way of recognising cues or indicators of resilience will be necessary. Separating resilience from success – process from outcome – will assist in clarifying the concept of resilience regardless of the outcome of an event. In other words, are there other abilities or activities that make a system resilient that can be identified separately from success or failure? There is a strong parallel here to system safety, since accidents can happen even in safe systems, and unsafe systems can operate for long periods without accidents.

There is a strong propensity to interpret and judge processes by their outcomes, as if the outcome validates (or not) a decision or action taken during the course of an event. This happens at several levels – expected outcomes generally require no explanation, while unexpected ones do. Since success (fortunately) is common, we habituate to it, and work leading to success thus becomes invisible, while work leading to failure, which is uncommon, receives detailed attention. It is often minutely analysed and in that process of reconstruction distorted, becoming a linear string of 'decisions' only distantly related to the reality of an event unfolding as a jumbled stream of perceptions and actions, bobs and weaves, ambiguous signals and shifting goals.

The bias created by this tendency can focus us in the wrong direction, leading to incorrect (albeit reassuring) conclusions about individuals, their actions, and the resilience of the system (Cook and Nemeth, 2010; Dekker, Nyce and Myers, 2012). Intellectually, it can be acknowledged that failure can occur in situations in which the best decisions possible were made based on the information to hand, and further that the converse is also true, that terrible decisions can be made but still result in success. Yet in post-incident assessments, judgements too often do not reflect this knowledge.

A manifestation of these conflicting positions can be seen in the common approach to managing acute chest pain in the emergency department. Because there is testing strategy that can distinguish life-threatening (e.g., heart attack) from benign (e.g., acid reflux) causes of chest pain, and because missing a heart attack risks substantial morbidity and mortality, emergency providers tend to be very risk averse in their management of all chest pain patients. Even though only a small proportion of chest pain cases are due to heart attacks or other life-threatening problems, all chest pain patients are initially viewed with concern, as if a heart attack were the cause, until proven otherwise. This means that most patients have a good outcome, even if the internal workings of the system lacked resilience along the way. But it would be a mistake to view this practice as resilient simply because the overwhelming majority of chest pain patients have a good outcome.

When Choosing the Right Action Removes the Rationale that Justified the Action Itself

A second problem that conflates resilience with success is that judicious actions sometimes appear unjustified in hindsight, because the evidence of their appropriateness is removed by their effectiveness. People add resilience to a system by having the experience, awareness, and judgement successfully to monitor, learn from, anticipate, and act upon non-routine situations

(Hollnagel, Woods and Leveson, 2006). Humans can often successfully anticipate and act on potential threats in order to forestall them. However, when such actions successfully remove the threat, this can often result in the threat becoming less obvious in hindsight, and the value of the preventative actions may therefore be under-appreciated. The actions might even appear dispensable, particularly when the threat was not discretely identifiable but was rather a drift towards failure (Dekker, 2011a).

A specific example of this can be seen in the well publicised death of a young boy due to sepsis, a day after he had been sent home from an emergency department (Dwyer, 2012). The emergency physician's alternative (and, in retrospect, preferable) choice would have been to admit the boy to the hospital, where he would have been put on intravenous antibiotics and closely observed. Multiple factors influenced the actions taken, such as the lack of available beds for admission, a difficult admitting physician who did not want to admit patients, resistance to admitting children who appear relatively well, pressures to reduce the 'unnecessary' use of antibiotics, antibiotic shortages, and others. These factors all affected the unfolding problem, but became invisible in hindsight. On the other hand, had the emergency physician admitted the patient, she would likely have been criticised for being too conservative and for misusing antibiotics, especially if the boy made an uneventful recovery. Here, the conflation of resilience with success risks falsely labelling resilient actions as superfluous and wasteful.

Case Studies

Let us consider two cases from health care in order to better explore the distinctions between resilience and success: the first with a bad outcome despite a resilient system ('failure in a resilient system'), and the other with a good outcome despite a non-resilient system ('success in a brittle system').

Case 1: Failure in a Resilient System

A 24-year-old sailor presented to the emergency department (ED) with three days of intermittent pain and numbness in his left leg, accompanied by recurrent short episodes of dizziness and low blood pressure. The emergency physician noticed that the patient had an unusual but characteristic deformity in his breastbone that is associated with a genetic predisposition for aortic dissection, a life-threatening disorder where the wall of the largest blood vessel in the body weakens and can rupture. The concern was deepened by a severely abnormal chest x-ray that made the diagnosis of aortic dissection highly likely in the physician's mind, and suggested that emergency surgery was needed. The emergency physician paged the cardiovascular surgery service (usually answered by a resident in training) but did not receive any response. She quickly escalated to paging the attending (supervising) cardiovascular surgeon on call and again did not receive a return call. Based on a hunch that perhaps the cardiovascular team was in the operating room, she turned to an unorthodox solution of calling the operating room (OR) directly, and indeed found that they were in the middle of an operation. She asked the OR nurse to open the patient's chest x-ray on the monitor in the operating room, recognising that this emergency case would be very disruptive, given that the team was in surgery, and anticipating that the strongly abnormal chest x-ray would be more persuasive than a verbal report. Based on this novel method for escalating an urgent case and need for surgical intervention, the cardiovascular surgeon prepared an emergency operating team. The patient was thus in the operating room shortly after arriving in the ED. However, approximately four hours into what was predicted to be an eight-hour surgical repair, the patient suffered a sudden cardiac arrest and could not be resuscitated, despite aggressive efforts.

This case illustrates resilient actions of anticipation and adaptation in response to an emergent need. (There was also some limited learning, in that the strategy of displaying a persuasive image in the OR has now become generalised.) The outcome, however, was the death of the patient, so the episode could be deemed a failure in a resilient system.

Case 2: Success in a Brittle System

The next case requires a bit of context about emergency departments (EDs) in the United States. EDs are often described at the 'front door' of any medical centre, as almost 50 per cent of hospital admissions originate in the ED (Schuur and Venkatesh, 2012). Thus, EDs contribute to the economic health of the organisation, since a hospital's primary revenue comes from admitted patients. Because of this, hospitals often compete on the basis of the apparent efficiency of their EDs. They track a number of 'throughput' factors in patients' ED visits, such as waiting time to see a doctor, and length of stay in the ED, because these factors are easily evident to patients and thus can provide a competitive advantage or disadvantage.

Because of new competition, a large, very busy ED decided to improve its throughput measures by changing its intake process for patients from the traditional nursing triage model to a physician-based 'rapid assessment' model. In traditional nurse triage, a patient is initially seen by a nurse who assigns a priority level that determines the order in which the patients are seen, based on the seriousness of their illness. For example, level 1 cases are seen immediately while level 5 cases can safely remain in the waiting room. However, this system delays the start of the patient's evaluation while they sit in the waiting room awaiting a physician examination. The new model supplanted the nurse-driven model and created a 'rapid assessment unit' (RAU), in which a physician performed the initial evaluation at the time of arrival for all incoming patients and launched the work-up and treatment plan for all those cases expected to take less than two hours for evaluation and treatment. After an eight-month trial, ED performance measures improved: patient satisfaction had increased from the 60th to 90th percentile, average patient wait time was decreased, the number leaving without being seen decreased, patient throughput had increased, and no adverse events were directly attributed to this new system. The programme was deemed a success based on these operational metrics. Of note, there were no predefined safety metrics when the system change was put into place.

Yet the staff assessment of the new RAU programme told a different story. Physicians and nurses working in the RAU reported feeling as if they were 'always working just on the edge'. The ED staff had a difficult time maintaining situational awareness due to lack of patient flow regulation leading to cognitive overload. They perceived that they had no safety margin, and that a single unexpected event or patient could put them into an unsafe and hazardous condition. Staff described dramatic increased stress levels, as they felt they were making 'snap' judgements without enough information. One staff member reported her work as 'just hoping for the best, trusting to luck.'

Work across the ED was noted to be disrupted in unanticipated ways, everything from electronic whiteboard status updates to ECGs not travelling with the patient. Many work processes that involved the larger macro system were impacted (radiology, lab, communications, admissions). There were increased interruptions from a new type of phone call that became necessary to transfer patients from the RAU to the main ED treatment areas. Scepticism and distrust emerged around the judgements made by practitioners who were working in the RAU. Reviews of some 'near miss' cases revealed failures to develop shared mental models for care for patients whose care originated within the RAU.

Case 2 demonstrates 'success in a brittle system' – an inability to anticipate the loss of adaptive capacity occasioned by the optimisation of the more 'routine' cases; a loss of resilience in the system with subsequent unanticipated consequences, despite 'success' as defined by the programme's target measures.

How Can the Separation of Resilience from Outcomes be Helpful to Health Care Organisations?

Separating resilience from outcome can help broaden understanding of failure beyond what is identified by root cause analyses of cases with bad outcomes. This could be helpful for two reasons. First, it can provide a lens for identifying events where the most significant contributing factors were system issues, rather than the judgements and decisions made by the human actors. Additionally it can highlight decisions made in the midst of failure that contributed positively to a bad situation, mitigating some aspects of the developing failure. These decisions might then be reinforced or emphasised. Second, the qualifying of outcomes could also change the way we look at successful events which are much more frequent but rarely analysed. This can help us understand (and emphasise) how a system overcame barriers to achieve success. Some cases may have successful outcomes despite the absence of resilience (success in a brittle system), and others may have unsuccessful outcome despite the presence of resilience (failure in a resilient system).

Case 1 demonstrates resilient behaviour not only by the emergency physician but also by the surgical team in the operating room. Members of the team, including the surgeon, were open to participating in an unorthodox method of consultation (a workaround) that deviated markedly from prescribed protocols for consultation and escalation. This is an important example of a workaround strategy contributing to resilience rather than having a negative impact on the system.

The importance of this may be difficult to appreciate until one considers the role of hierarchy within complex adaptive microsystems such as a surgical team. In health care, consultation protocols for 'on-call care' provide a mechanism for managing unscheduled disruptions to work. We know that in complex adaptive systems, expert and experienced workers continually develop adaptations to new or unrecognised constraints (in Case 1, the emergency physician was faced with an inability to obtain emergent surgical consultation for a critical patient, an unusual event). These adaptations, a form of workaround strategies, are an example of resilience. Adaptive workarounds may make the system safer, as in Case 1. The qualification of outcomes as seen in Figure 13.1 could provide an opportunity for adaptive workarounds to be recognised as sources of rescue and recovery from inadequately designed systems rather than deemed willful acts of non-compliance by health care administrations and regulatory agencies.

Case 2, an example of success in a brittle system, highlights the importance of anticipating and monitoring for unintended consequences of interventions for the sake of increasing economic efficiency. Health care organisations have recently become fascinated with normalising operations, using methods such as six-sigma, Lean, practice guidelines, quality improvement, the Toyota production system, and others. Attempts to protocolise simple and complicated systems such as assembly lines and other linear processes may be successful. However, it has long been recognised (at least in other domains) that such solutions can be ineffective or even counterproductive when applied indiscriminately to situations for which they are not suited,

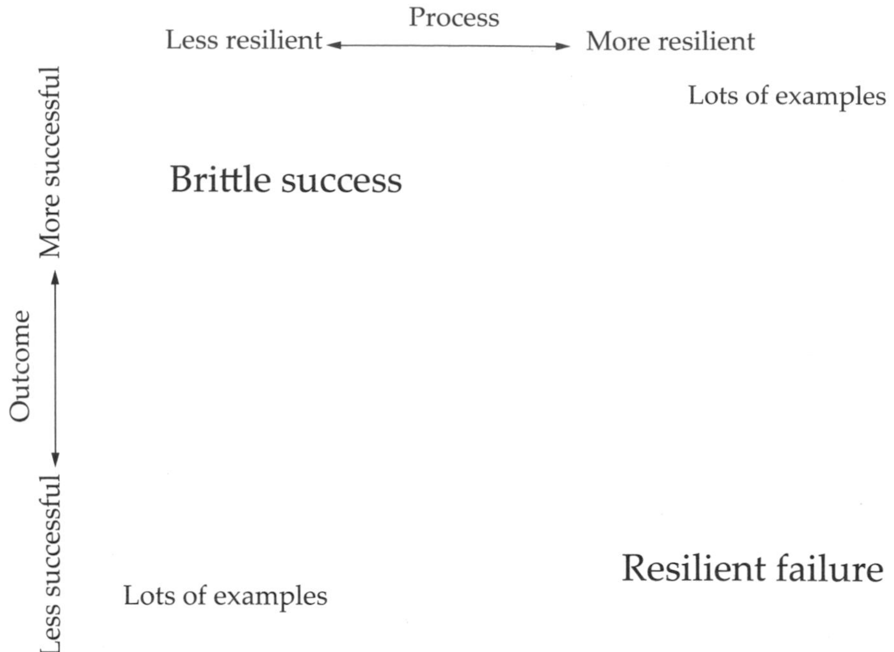

Figure 13.1 The separation of resilience from outcome. Some cases may have successful outcomes despite the absence of resilience (success in a brittle system), and others may have unsuccessful outcome despite the presence of resilience (failure in a resilient system)

such as complex systems (Hayes and Wheelwrite, 1979a; Hayes and Wheelwrite, 1979b; Perrow, 1967; Reason, 1997). There are certainly some linear forms of optimisations that improve some aspects of work, such as increasing patient satisfaction by shortening wait times, but the new procedures introduced in Case 2 also reduced the workers' ability to adapt in a resilient fashion.

In Case 2, one might also argue that there was a lack of resilience both in the RAU-EDs and in the organisation as a whole (or in the management layer). Resilience was lacking because there was no anticipation of the outcome, i.e., the increasing brittleness. Consequences of change are classically believed to be readily apparent, but as illustrated here, they can be delayed or opaque as a consequence of the normal margins for safety being undermined. The qualification of 'success' in this case in terms of resilience provides an opportunity to elucidate the 'hard to see' consequences of change upon safety.

Conclusion

Success and resilience should be treated as two different orthogonal dimensions of performance. Health professionals already are familiar with the distinction between process and outcome, but they are vulnerable to the conflation of the two, especially in the light of regulatory and organisational messaging that emphasises 'compliance' with policy and procedures for improved clinical outcomes. Maintaining a clear separation of process and outcome, and restricting the notion of resilience to a system's processes (i.e., what the system does), should help care delivery organisations avoid the sorts of narrow optimisations that can reduce small common problems at the price of increasing large, rare ones. It should also help move the organisation's focus from a Safety-I perspective (if nothing went wrong, then everything must be alright, and vice versa) to a Safety-II perspective where the organisation monitors not only its output, but also its capacity to respond, monitor, learn, and anticipate.

Chapter 14
Adaptation versus Standardisation in Patient Safety

Sheuwen Chuang

Introduction

Most patient safety systems train health care staff using standardised procedures or guidelines. Although these trainees gain skill in acting according to standard procedures that potentially benefit patient safety, health care systems are dynamic; their components (physicians, managers, patients) and external conditions are always changing. Undesired events occur when safety systems cannot help health care organisations and staff adapt to changing situations.

Three scabies outbreaks during a 17-month period in the respiratory care wards of a Taiwan hospital (Chuang, 2012; Chuang, Howley and Lin, 2011) illustrate how standardised procedures failed to stop worsening outbreaks from recurring. The hospital has faced expanding costs in providing respiratory care services under the global budget of the national health insurance scheme, and these outbreaks occurred in a context of increasing numbers of patients on prolonged mechanical ventilation in the last ten years. During the 17-month period infection density increased from 0.38 per cent to 1.59 per cent to 2.07 per cent. During each scabies outbreak, in addition to confirming the diagnosis and initiating immediate medical treatment, a task force investigated each outbreak using root cause analysis.

The major root cause in the first outbreak was found to be that there was no standard procedure for checking visitors' skin conditions, so the ward established a self-declaration form and reporting procedure for visitors. After 270 days, the second outbreak occurred. It centred on a patient who was suspected to be infected with scabies, but who lacked a confirmed diagnosis and had been housed in a general ward. As the doctor in charge adhered to the standard procedure (no isolation without confirmation of scabies), this time the corrective action was to add a rule under which patients who are suspected of having scabies can be isolated for two weeks and treated with anti-scabies medicine.

Six months later, the third scabies outbreak occurred when a patient with a scabies-like condition was isolated for two weeks, but then moved back to a general ward because a diagnosis of scabies was not yet confirmed. Later the patient was found to have crusted scabies, but the doctor in charge adhered to the guideline that a patient could only be isolated for up to 14 days if scabies was not confirmed at the end of the isolation. These three scabies outbreaks illustrate health care workers' typical reactions in dealing with safety incidents: when something happens, people deal with each case alone and react rather than think ahead.

Several issues raised by standardisation are revealed in this example. First, it is clear that although people expect policies and procedures to ensure patient safety, this is not always the case. Second, cost concerns can dominate standardisation decisions. A third issue is that following standardised rules reduces the need for communication and collaboration among clinicians. Fourth, current safety systems using root cause analysis did not improve safety in this case. All health care organisations face these four issues, because standardisation cannot always succeed in ensuring patient safety. To prevent future errors, it is not enough to learn from failures (as in root cause analysis) and to standardise what is learned.

Building system resilience is a better way of coping with rapid and unexpected changes as well as time and resource pressures in health care. Resilience in this case is learning and adapting to create safety in settings fraught with gaps, hazards, trade-offs and multiple goals (Cook, Render and Woods, 2000). This chapter discusses how organisational and individual standardisation and adaptation behaviours shape safety strategy and planning. On a more practical level, recommendations are made for several ways that patient safety issues can be analysed from a resilience perspective.

Inherent Operational Safety Problems

Health care organisations use policies and guidelines to standardise and clarify care routines in order to improve efficiency, productivity and safety. Health care staff are expected to comply with and keep up to date with numerous policies covering their daily work. This work-as-imagined is what designers, managers, regulators and authorities believe happens or should happen. In some situations, staff follow or even persist with these rules. However, because work and change occur rapidly and unexpectedly in a continuous stream, employees may for various reasons break, modify, work around or implement these rules inconsistently. This process of compromise between work-as-imagined and actual novel situations leads to endless small-scale events that aggregate to constitute everyday work performance.

A systematic review attempts to synthesise research findings into a defensible case of what is known about a given topic, then typically discusses what remains unknown and what should be done about the findings to date. A recent systematic review associated preventable harm in health care primarily with situations in which: (1) an identifiable, modifiable cause was present (44 per cent); (2) reasonable adaptation to a process would prevent future recurrences (23 per cent); and (3) guidelines were not followed (16 per cent) (Nabhan et al., 2012). That study contributed a quantitative recognition that prevention of harm can be achieved primarily through the three critical themes. All of this could be disputed based on a resilience orientation and Safety-II thinking, which argues that it is better to focus on where and how things go right than where and how they go wrong. The first of the above points would tend to be rejected by Safety-II adherents. The second and third situations in particular imply that in addition to standardisation, reasonable adaptation to processes is important for patient safety. The third situation presumes that an existing guideline applied to the given situation and, if followed correctly, should prevent harm associated with care.

Situations (2) and (3) represent types of operational problems in patient safety: under-adaptation failure and non-compliance with policies and procedures. These problems are inherent in health systems and make undesirable events inevitable.

Under-adaptation Failure

Under-adaptation failure occurs when people persist in applying standardised work procedures or activities in the face of evidence that changing circumstances demand a qualitative shift in assessment, priorities or response (Woods, 2006). In retrospect, it is clear that the three scabies outbreaks represent this kind of failure. Similar cases of under-adaptation are found where automation is introduced in areas such as robotic surgery (Chapter 8). Such cases lead to an ironic situation where automation erodes critical manual control skills that are still needed in case the job cannot be done via automation (Dekker et al., 2008).

Following the 'rules' for decision making or interactions does not require negotiation. Rules offer a quick, safe (for decision makers) and cost-reducing course of action (Patterson, 2008). Failures caused by following standards therefore are treated as system errors requiring new or changed operational procedures instead of being recognised as lack of staff adaptability. In a study of root cause analysis in health care, Card, Ward and Clarkson (2011) found administrative controls were the most commonly recommended and implemented activities (80 per cent of corrective actions) after root cause analysis. These administrative controls included establishment and refinement of policies, procedures and training. Yet in the rapidly changing environment of health care, it is unrealistic to look at the future only in light of the past and to expect standard procedures to prevent future failures.

The conventional improvement cycles have been dominated by the concept of Safety-I and the plan-do-check-act (PDCA) model for decades, resulting in the occurrences of undesirable events due to under-adaptation and non-compliance. The following sections explain how this concept and approach govern improvements in patient safety.

Non-compliance with Policies and Procedures

Organisations establish standards, policies and procedures to set performance expectations and promote accountability for meeting these expectations. In practice, the increment of non-compliance with standards and policies has been a concern. Carthey et al. (2011) argued that large numbers of guidelines from many different sources make it impossible for staff to comply with all of them. Hollnagel (2004) lists four conditions usually assumed in planning work situations: inputs to the work process are regular and predictable, work demands and resources are within limits, working conditions generally fall within normal limits, and output complies with expectations or norms. Yet work-as-done indicates that these four conditions are often not fulfilled. Health care workers adjust their work practices to get the job done because of insufficient time or resources. They also optimise non-compliance for company or personal benefit, or find official procedures difficult to follow under specific and novel circumstances (cf. Chapter 1).

As handovers in all health care settings are highly variable in content and process, they are frequently an area of non-compliance with standards and procedures. To avoid such errors and prevent harm, the World Health Organisation (2007) suggests a standardised approach to handover communication between staff at changes of shift and between different care units during patient transfers. However, most handovers do not occur under ideal conditions, and staff often lack time to transfer patient data appropriately (Raduma-Tomàs et al., 2011). Because humans are adaptable and tend to improvise, non-compliances in handovers are inevitable (Amalberti et. al., 2006); thus handover-related incidents are frequently found in malpractice claims (Hoffman, 2007; Andrews and Millar, 2005).

Non-compliance with policies and procedures represents a certain level of adaptation to a situation for various reasons. Whether people intend to follow the rules or not, standardisation cannot address all situations in complex health care system.

And as Patterson (2008) noted, imposing a simple standard on a complex process does not result in simplicity. Well-intentioned standardisation cannot suffice for patient safety, and widespread non-compliance with health care standards and policies renders these protections suboptimal as well.

Current Improvement Methodology

Health care systems require continuous improvement and adaptation. Figure 14.1 illustrates the conventional systems development approach to patient safety. Initially, every system has a pre-established competence that models how strategies and countermeasures handle variability and uncertainties in daily work. However, as each day brings disturbances from within or outside the system (such as new demands, pressures on time and resources, and other surprises), health care organisation and staff competence may be incomplete, limited or inappropriate. All of these undermine the effectiveness of the system, producing unsatisfactory patient safety outcomes through its inherent operational problems, under-adaptation and non-compliance; these undesirable outcomes activate an improvement cycle that revises the 'as-is' system. And this kind of improvement is repeated over and over again.

Patient Safety Indicators

Patient safety indicators (PSIs) are administrative quality measures that focus on in-hospital events associated with preventable harms during care (Agency for Healthcare Research and Quality, 2008). PSIs are intended to raise awareness of harm and can be collected from direct observation, medical records, administrative data, malpractice claims, and reporting of errors, near misses, and adverse events. Although there is still no international consensus on patient safety indicators (Chang et al., 2005), McLoughlin et al. (2006) noted that awareness of harm emerged particularly in five domains: hospital-acquired infections, operative and post-operative complications, sentinel events, obstetrics and other care-related events such as falls. These indicators can be classified in two categories. *Sentinel indicators* identify individual events or phenomena that are intrinsically undesirable, such as wrong-site surgery or medication errors; this information is collected through incident reporting. *Rate-based indicators* use data about events that are expected to occur with some frequency. These can be expressed as proportions or rates (such as hospital-acquired infections) derived from data collected from incident reporting, administrative records or periodic auditing (Mainz, 2003; McLoughlin et al., 2006).

Figure 14.1 presents unsatisfied patient safety outcomes in these two categories. The sentinel indicators are displayed as a triangle with the inference of 1-10-30-600 ratio based on the Bird theory positing 630 no-injury incidents, for every ten minor and one major (serious) injury accidents. In this category, adverse events represent the extreme of poor performance, and they generally trigger further investigation using root cause analysis.

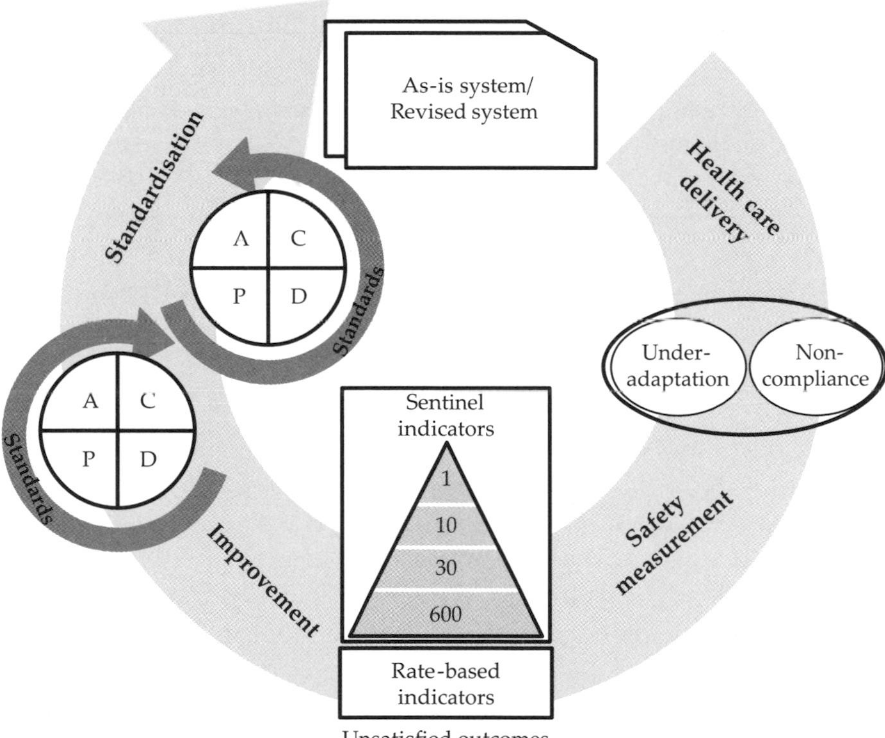

Figure 14.1 Conventional systems development approach to patient safety

The rate-based indicators represent adverse safety outcomes of high occurrence but low or medium severity, such as hospital-acquired infections. Because it is difficult to define a salient event, this category does not map into a clear incident for investigation. As the magnitude of harm involved may be insufficient as a serious safety issue for immediate remediation by health care organisations and staff, quality improvement methods such as quality circles or team resource management are often applied to this category of patient safety issues. Both root cause analysis and other quality improvement activities undertaken by health care organisations are widely believed to have prophylactic effects (Greenberg, 2010).

Patient safety has been measured typically by the above two 'after-the-fact' types of measurements. These 'lagging' indicators, which provide historical information about patient safety, raise the awareness of harm. However, an essential purpose in measuring safety is to develop intervention strategies to avoid future accidents. With lagging indicators, any changes made may influence future performance but cannot alter the outcome of these incidents (Grabowski et al., 2007). On the other hand, safety professionals recognise that noting signals before an accident occurs offers potential opportunities to improve safety (Grabowski et al., 2007; Rivard, Rosen and Carroll, 2006). These leading indicators, which are one type of accident precursor, can include certain conditions, events or measures that precede an undesirable event and that have some value in predicting such events. Therefore, using process measures of health care quality as leading indicators is suggested because they are more sensitive than outcome measures, and are likely to be more actionable, in that they are easier to interpret (Mant and Hicks, 1995; Mant, 2001). In addition to process measures, Rivard et al. (2006) argued that near-miss data assist timely organisational learning because they may act more as leading indicators compared with adverse event data. Using leading indicators has the advantage that actions can be taken to alter the course of patient safety performance.

Learning from Failures and the PDCA Cycle

Hollnagel (2012) defines Safety-I as a condition where the number of adverse outcomes (accidents / incidents / near-misses) is as low as possible. In one sense, this definition directs our efforts to search for safety problems only where things have already gone wrong, whether or not the outcome was preventable (Henriksen and Kaplan, 2003), and then to improve system safety through past experiences and analysis of what went wrong. These methods for learning from failures, such as root cause analysis and quality improvement activities, focus on what has gone wrong and / or what has low safety performance, and are used to find causes leading to wrong acts or behaviours and to recommend corrective actions.

The plan-do-check-act (PDCA) cycle is a popular approach used for industrial quality improvement activities (Moen and Norman, 2012; Tague, 2004). This includes planning (definition of problem and hypothesis about possible causes and solutions), doing (implementing), checking (evaluating results) and acting (returning to planning stage if results are unsatisfactory, or standardising results if satisfactory). Regulators and managers demand, or request, compliance with new standards. As shown in Figure 14.1, the PDCA cycle generates new rules or guidelines (standards) which are added to the 'as-is' system model for the purpose of system improvement. The conventional logic of PDCA features heavily in the patient safety systems development cycle.

Safety-I leads health care staff to react to unsatisfactory outcomes that are mostly caused by the system's inherent operational problems. In the PDCA cycle, safety improvements emphasise prevention of error recurrence by establishing standards based on successful corrective actions. This overall approach of learning from failures and seeking safety via standardisation, as shown in Figure 14.1, develops in an incremental manner: the tried and trusted procedures are only changed when they fail, and then usually by adding one more request or element (an updated or new rule). Thus the unintended consequence of having too many rules can be expected.

Despite the value of this approach for both individual and organisational learning, its effectiveness is limited, as when recommended actions are not fully integrated into the relevant organisational structure (Kuhn and Youngberg, 2002). Such methods do not support health care workers in generating more robust risk control plans (Wu, Lipshutz and Pronovost, 2008;

Pham et al., 2010). As only the most serious safety events trigger root cause analysis to learn from failures, opportunities for learning may be insufficient. The PDCA cycle and quality improvement activities potentially reinforce people's belief in standardisation for safety. Yet as noted above, conventional patient safety approaches such as root cause analysis, quality management activities, standardisation and more procedures can erode health care organisations' and staff members' adaptability and ability to anticipate risks before harm occurs.

Resilience as a Safety Philosophy

Resilience engineering represents a new way of thinking about safety that addresses the deficits of conventional approaches. To apply standardisation and adaptation adequately in dealing with dynamic health care systems, resilience researchers have urged several changes in the philosophy of safety management. These are:

- Making sure that things go right as much as possible (Safety-II), rather than emphasising negative outcomes of care and following habitual acts persistently. Safety-II means focusing on processes rather than outcomes and proactively adjusting performance for everyday work success (Hollnagel, 2012).
- Recognising that performance variability is inevitable in daily work. While standardisation is implemented in a PDCA cycle, the concept of performance variability can be used in the process. Standardisation provides an opportunity to restructure how patient safety work is normatively conducted; the concept brings flexible thinking within the revising structure to tailor the plan to specific contexts, support exception handling for non-routine cases, and enable adaptation to feedback about priorities when making trade-offs.

Innovative Methods

In addition to philosophy changes, Chuang and Howley's (2012) enriched system-oriented events analysis (SOEA) model suggests the methodology listed below for analysis of patient safety issues.

System Analysis Supplants Root Cause Analysis

Health care is a complex dynamic system where most events result from a non-linear network structure of system flows, and where errors may arise from many combinations of systemic conditions. Root cause analysis uncovers systems-level causes and contributing factors behind incidents (factor thinking) and eliminates causes by disabling possible cause–effect links (linear thinking). This method fails to address the systemic nature of problems, and consequently it is difficult to build system resilience without understanding the whole system. SOEA adopts systems thinking to event analysis by providing a formulated procedure and relevant instruments to examine system factors or elements while evaluating the whole structure of the targeted system. Resilience engineering methods depend on users comprehending the whole system to understand interactions between system components, as compared with root cause analysis focusing on investigations of linear cause and effect.

Learn from High-frequency Multi-events

Safety-I emphasises learning from failures, yet health care regulations generally require root cause analysis only in the case of adverse events or sentinel events with high severity but low frequency (World Alliance for Patient Safety, 2005). A broader group of incidents with higher occurrences (unintended events) including near-misses, no-harm errors and events with lower severity codes are generally analysed using descriptive statistics to reflect frequencies or they are examined at health care managers' discretion (Braithwaite et al., 2006). Without appropriate analysis of these incidents and feedback to clinical systems, significant opportunities are missed to identify, learn about and correct system weaknesses before tragedy occurs.

In the Safety-II perspective, learning from past experiences involves three conditions: (1) opportunity to learn (learning situations or cases must be frequent enough for a learning practice to develop); (2) sufficient similarity (learning situations must have enough in common to allow for generalisation); and (3) opportunity to verify (it must be possible to verify that the learning was 'correct' via feedback) (Hollnagel, 2012). As unintended incidents frequently indicate deeper underlying problems of everyday performance, small improvements of these incidents may provide more benefit than a large improvement in exceptional performance. Analysing a number of frequent and similar incidents thoroughly is probably more valuable than a cursory overview of a large number of incidents. The SOEA model provides an integrated platform which can support the investigation of multiple events at one time and allows unintended events to be efficiently analysed.

Alignment of Risk Controls across Organisational Levels

Rasmussen (1997) argued that without coordinated change at various levels of a socio-technical system, external forces acting on the system may unintentionally '[prepare] the stage for an accident.' To prevent undesirable events, risk controls must be finalised and fully integrated into the organisation. Risk control aims to achieve particular behaviours to maintain conditions for desired levels of patient safety. The root causes of safety failure can be seen as control flaws (inadequate control or no control) behind identified hazards. However, this view disguises the systemic nature of required controls, as these are often not accessible via root cause analysis alone. SOEA provides a method of risk alignment across organisational levels allowing investigators and practitioners to focus on critical interrelationships across the whole system.

Conclusion

Although the Taiwan hospital followed standards persistently and applied root cause analysis in linear thinking as the strategy for patient safety, it experienced recurring scabies outbreaks. Since the hospital tried enriched system-oriented events analysis (SOEA) to re-analyse and act on the third scabies outbreak, no nosocomial scabies infections were reported for more than 1,161 days. SOEA's distinctive capabilities exceed those of root cause analysis in systems analysis, multiple events analysis, and risk control formulation and alignment. In the Taiwan case, SOEA helped control a scabies problem where root cause analysis had not. This example provides several lessons for improving patient safety:

- Root cause analysis and similar methods that look for fragmented causes, especially at operational levels, overlook organisational factors and fail to develop collaboration across departments and organisational levels to prevent future undesirable events.
- Adaptation requires collaboration between clinicians. Doctors, nurses and support staff share responsibility in detecting and acting on threats such as scabies.
- As SOEA leads to system adaptation, it creates a common ground for understanding interactions between system components, and encourages collaboration between clinicians based on its philosophical commitment to system analysis. Effective system analysis requires an understanding of underlying structures and processes rather than events.
- While standardisation is important, the plan-do-check-act cycle cannot suffice to revise pre-developed competence models based on past experiences (learning from failures). Staff developed compromised actions to handle temporary isolations for suspected scabies patients based on the understanding of interdependences and interactions between clinicians through the SOEA systems analysis. Safety planners should encourage an adjustment-friendly attitude to support handling of exceptions in non-routine cases and to enable adaptation to feedback when making trade-offs.

Chapter 15
The Use of PROMs to Promote Patient Empowerment and Improve Resilience in Health Care Systems

Alessandra Gorini, Ketti Mazzocco and Gabriella Pravettoni

Shared Decision Making and Patient Empowerment

In recent years there have been significant moves to attempt to transform the traditional paternalistic approach, in which the physicians are parental, recommending what they feel is best for the patient, to an informative, patient-centered approach. Such an approach assumes that the physician should inform and discuss with the patients all available treatment choices, helping them to choose their preferred treatment option. The patient-centered approach considers it essential for the patient to be actively involved and to participate in the decision making processes concerning treatment in order to ensure that decisions are consistent with the patient's values, preferences and needs.

Shared decision making aligned with patient-centered medicine involves a bi-directional information exchange and joint agreement between the physician and the patient (Neuman, Charlson and Temple, 2007). For shared decision making to be effective, the content of communication in a medical consultation should include both factual data and the patient's considerations. While the former is derived from the physician's knowledge, medical information and clinical tools, the latter is provided directly by the patient, who has personal experience of the illness, its symptoms, its effects on her everyday experiences and quality of life. 'In an ideal world …' Barnato et al. (2007: 627) stated, 'patients would come to a medical consultation armed with sufficient knowledge, clarity about their personal value, and the ability to engage in a thoughtful discussion about the pros and cons of treatment options. Providers, in turn, would be prepared to support their patients, armed with an understanding of the patient's knowledge gaps, personal values about possible outcomes and treatment preferences.' However, clinical consultations usually take place under conditions of limited time and resources, where the physician's talk overwhelms the patient's preferences and considerations.

This gap between optimal conditions and many actual encounters could be reduced by implementing specific instruments to assess the so-called patient-reported outcome measures (PROMs). PROMs can be defined as 'reports coming directly from patients about how they function or feel in relation to a health condition and its therapy, without interpretation of the patients' responses by physician or anyone else' (Valderas, Alonso and Guyatt, 2008). Such measures are thus instruments that provide patient-based information about health, illness and the effects of treatment as inputs into decisions.

Addressing the rationale behind quality of life assessment in the clinical context, the use of PROMs is reasoned to benefit patient care in multiple ways. First, it increases physicians' and nurses' awareness of patients' perspectives on their condition and previous inputs into their health-related quality of life, thereby easing the discussion of these aspects. Second, it has the potential to identify and prioritise physical or psychosocial problems that otherwise might have been overlooked or remain unrecognised. Since these problems might affect how patients are treated, their detection is essential. Third, the patients' preferences for specific outcome goals can be identified. This is important because physicians' and patients' priorities often differ, sometimes substantially, concerning the aims of treatment, the impact of the disease on patients' lives and the values of possible outcomes. Additionally, the incorporation of patients' preferences enables an anticipation of benefits regarding their adherence to treatment. Fourth, PROMs allow for the monitoring of disease progression and treatment that may not be revealed via clinical testing. Fifth, PROMs can be used as screening instruments investigating unmet needs that require referral. Sixth, as a result of including PROMs in the treatment process, the patient might feel better cared for, which could positively influence their emotional functioning. And last, but most important, PROMs in clinical practice have been found to facilitate and improve communication between the physician and the patient (Meadows, 2011, Greenhalgh et al., 2012). Despite the interconnectedness of these advantages, improved communication and heightened awareness of the patient's quality of life on the part of the physician is thought to be a key factor to improving the quality of care.

In general, a PROMS approach is reasoned to promote shared decision making and patient empowerment, which, in turn, should enhance individual resilience and consequently affect patients' outcomes. By fostering a shared decision making process and by generally empowering patients, increasing their chances of becoming more competent in making their own well-informed choices concerning the treatment, using PROMs in clinical practice is meant to improve delivery of care, lead to better patient outcomes manifested by reduced symptoms, and improve health-related quality of life and patient satisfaction.

Individual Resilience as a Result of Shared Decision Making

Just as shared decision making is a dynamic process that involves the interaction between professionals and patients, resilience can also be considered as a dynamic interaction between the individuals and their environment (Masten and Write, 2010), where the environment implies all who are involved in the patient's life, including the professionals who are part of the patient's decision making process. The similarity between shared decision making and resilience (both being processes that require interaction among people), makes the former a fertile field of inspiration for the latter, showing how the whole system plays an important role in affecting resilience: individual attributes, family aspects, social environment, professionals and institutions (Ungar, 2006, 2008).

In a health care context, where clinicians and patients interact for relatively short periods of time, it might be challenging, but nevertheless crucial, to understand all the factors that enhance the probability of recovery from adverse events, starting, possibly, with the patient. In other words, while investigating resilience in the health care system, we cannot ignore individual resilience. Indeed, the only people who see the whole picture of the patient's journey are the patients themselves.

From a psychological perspective, individual resilience can be defined as the ability to utilise resources to cope with adversity. Different studies have come up with different ways of categorising such resources (e.g., Kumpfer 1999; McWhiter et al., 2007). Grothberg (1995) proposes to group the sources of resilience in (1) external support (family, friends, communities, etc.); (2) internal strength (feelings, attitudes, values); and (3) interpersonal skills (communication, problem solving, management of feelings and temperament, social relationships).

Grothberg's categorisation seems to fit well within the 'shared decision making–empowerment' process, where even modest personal control over their destinies will help people persist in mastering tasks and become more committed to making positive life changes and where choice, in this perspective, becomes essential to motivate changes (Bender et al., 2007). Converging with Bender and colleagues' views, resources of resilience can be identified in the personal sense of competence, self-efficacy, sense of agency, health beliefs and self-reliance (Hass and Graydon, 2009; Maluccio, 2002), all factors that involve the freedom and ability to make choices. In addition, a critical role in fostering individual resilience seems to be found in the patient's emotions. While negative emotions are detrimental, positive emotions can not only make robust contributions toward resilience, but can also be effectively cultivated. That, in turn, will tend to advance skills to enhance health, resilience, and wellbeing (Fredrickson, 2002; Fredrickson et al., 2003).

When facing an adverse event, the personal resilient resources previously described may be at risk of decreasing, while cognitive demands on the patient may increase. Imagine, for example, a person who has just been diagnosed with a cancer. Negative emotional reactions can occur such as depression and anxiety, fear caused by uncertainty about the future, and a perception of lack of control over what is happening. Associated with physical problems such as pain and fatigue, the patient might need to change their plans and often reorganise their life around the illness. These factors can be viewed as a decrease in the capacity to cope with the adverse event. In other words, the weight in the balance between demands on the person and the resources available to her favors the demands. Engaging with the challenging event becomes critical and may increase the probability of negative outcomes. Such an engagement to cope can occur 'naturally' (where the patient relies on individual resources, when personality and cognitive factors remain robust) or it may be fostered by some type of intervention, in which the individual is empowered to acquire a sense of control over her behavior, feelings, and thoughts (O'Leary and Bhaju, 2006).

The interaction between patients and clinicians may be a key context in which this intervention might be performed. A better understanding of patients' needs, through the use of PROMs, is fundamental to guide the delivery of effective information to the patients and to support the shared decision making process that, in turn, helps increase individual resilience.

The Role of Patient Empowerment to Increase Resilience in the Health Care System

Other than increasing personal patients' resilience, giving them the possibility of becoming active participants in the therapeutic process, the whole 'shared decision making–empowerment process' can also contribute to increase the resilience in the health care system in general.

There is an increasing tendency for patients to complain or mobilise malpractice claims against health care providers when things go wrong. This is mainly due to two reasons: when poor quality of care is experienced, or when patients are not allowed or are unable to participate in medical decisions by expressing their opinions and preferences. Medical malpractice claims represent a serious economic problem for health care organisations, significantly increasing their direct costs (i.e. insurance premiums) and indirect costs (i.e. increasing the practice of defensive medicine). In line with what we have discussed, Cassel and Guest (2012) recently suggested that shared decision making would help reduce this waste of money, and the poor quality care affecting the US health care system. They argued that 'a major goal of health care reform is enhancing patient-centered care', improving patient–physician communication, patient engagement in clinical decision making, quality, and access to medical information and care.

Empowering patients to increase their awareness of the benefits of, and their motivation for, engaging in informed choices can become of crucial importance to help health care providers take into account not only the patient's quantity of life (that is, in general, an objective variable with the same value for patients, physicians, policymakers and researchers). In fact, even the patient's quality of life may be evaluated very differently by the patient and the physician. In conclusion, we argue that understanding the subjective evaluation of quality of life may become of primary importance to improve patients' satisfaction about the treatment they receive, consequently increasing the general resilience of health care systems.

Conclusion

When a person is affected by an illness, the question of how possible treatments or interventions will affect the individual often becomes an open experiment for the two co-investigators – the patient and the physician (and, more broadly, the entire health care system). A dynamic journey begins, especially in the case of long-term diseases. In such cases, it is crucial to ensure the patient is an active agent in this dynamic journey, in order to enhance the probability of positive outcomes. These can be translated into recovery (or at least improvement in the quality of life) for the patient, and, hopefully, lower costs for the entire health system.

It thus becomes of great importance to develop an intervention (such as the use of PROMs) to activate the 'shared decision-making–empowerment' process, where the physician offers the best possible options for curing the patient and where patients understand clearly what they are dealing with and can decide how to approach the challenges, and often devastating experiences. The goal is increased resilience, starting at the very beginning of the physician–patient encounter.

Chapter 16
Resilient Health Care

Rob Robson

The underlying assumption for this chapter posits a close link between the type of system in which the event being reviewed has occurred, the type of analytic approach that is most likely to be helpful and the way in which safety investigators can be most effectively trained. There will also be brief consideration of the various types of investigation approaches, in order to determine which may be the most appropriate for a given system.

Learning: An Essential Capability of a Resilient Organisation

The four elements or capabilities (Hollnagel, 2011b) that have been identified as necessary for an organisation to be resilient (*responding, monitoring, learning* and *anticipating*) are inter-related and interdependent. It is not helpful to speculate about the 'primacy' of one capability over another. At the same time, it is hard to imagine any of the capabilities being operational without significant *learning* having taken place and without a systematic link with the other elements of a resilient organisation.

Indeed, this concept has been elevated almost to the level of a mantra for many safety management system designers and managers in terms of the ability of organisations to prevent accidents through 'organizational learning from incidents' (Sanne, 2008).

Learning, it seems, is an essential quality of a resilient complex adaptive socio-technical system. More to the point, having a well developed system to promote *effective learning* on an ongoing basis is vital to the resilience efforts of such an organisation. It seems, therefore, useful to reflect on how to approach the development of such a learning system and how to train safety practitioners to apply effectively the principles and tools that are most adapted to the type of system in which events and incidents are occurring.

Reviewing Events as a Means to Promote Learning

As noted above (Sanne, 2008), there is support in the system safety community for the notion that reviewing and investigating a variety of occurrences, critical incidents and other harm events will lead to learning and in turn to a reduction of the risk of recurrence in the future. The retrospective review or investigation of 'things that have gone wrong' is extremely common in the system safety field. This approach reflects a fairly 'pure' Safety-I perspective and is motivated in the health care field at least in part by the view that the level of unintentional harm is unacceptable, compared to that seen in other complex socio-technical systems.

Safety-I thinking encounters major challenges in the form of abysmally low levels of reporting of events (and, in health care in particular, critical incidents involving significant harm to patients) coupled with organisational cultures which are perceived as being punitive in nature and which provide negative motivation for reporting. And there is a very real problem of inadequate resources that are (not) made available for system safety practitioners to undertake effective reviews that might promote organisational learning.

All in all, while many system safety practitioners believe that reviewing and investigating events leads to learning, and that learning will reduce the risk of future incidents (in spite of thin evidence to support such leaps of faith) there are many practical reasons why this particular application of Safety-I has not yet yielded obvious positive results.

One of the reasons why retrospective reviews of safety events in health care have not often produced recommendations leading to sustainable improvements in care processes clearly relates to the type of approach that is adopted. There is often a mismatch between the analytic method that is selected and the type of situation under review. Hollnagel (2004, 2012) has reviewed, both historically and functionally, the main types of approaches that have been developed to review critical incidents.

The approaches are differentiated on the basis of two main issues. The first relates to the method's view of causation (whether a traditional linear versus a non-linear approach is incorporated into the analytic method). The second issue concerns whether the approach assumes that the event can be viewed in relative isolation or needs to be viewed systemically, as an integral part of a complex adaptive socio-technical system. Hollnagel's analysis (2004) leads to the proposal that there are three main categories of retrospective safety event review:

1. Simple linear review methods – the common example is Heinrich's domino theory developed in the 1930s (Heinrich, 1931).
2. Complex / complicated linear review methods – exemplified by the 'Swiss cheese' model of Reason (1997).
3. Systemic non-linear approaches – a good example of such an approach is the functional resonance analysis method or FRAM (Hollnagel, 2012).

It is beyond the scope of this chapter to attempt a detailed description of the three approaches or an evaluation of the strengths and weaknesses of representative methods. A persuasive analysis of the weaknesses of linear approaches was undertaken by Dekker, Cilliers and Hofmeyr (2011). Lundberg and colleagues (2009) examined the manuals describing and analysing the investigation methods used in eight different Swedish safety domains, according to various criteria. Of interest is the fact that all methods examined were of the complex / complicated linear variety. The authors conclude that the various methods seem to reflect a newly enunciated principle – what-you-find-(in your investigation)-is-what-you-fix (WYFIWYF) – a somewhat less noble conclusion than that suggested by the earlier mentioned mantra of preventing accidents 'through organizational learning from incidents' (Sanne, 2008). The new proposed acronym is absolutely not to be confused with what-you-look-for-is-what-you-find (WYLFIWYF) – an observation by Hollnagel (2004) that characterises all approaches to the investigation and analysis of adverse events.

What Kind of System Are We Studying? Is Health Care so 'Different'?

There has been relatively little study of health care as a system, with a few notable exceptions. The idea of differentiating complicated from complex processes and systems was suggested by Plsek, who also contributed to a major review of the implications for health care of being a complex adaptive system (Zimmerman, Lindberg and Plsek, 1998).[1] The work of Kernick (2004), as well as that of Letiche (2008), provides descriptions of efforts to understand health care as a complex adaptive system (CAS). Nevertheless, health care 'exceptionalism' has largely insulated researchers, planners, managers and providers from looking at other complex systems for guidance.[2]

The lack of attention to the nature of health care as a complex system is not restricted to health care itself. One of the early seminal works on complex organisations (Perrow, 1999) used a four-quadrant grid created by the axes of *coupling* (tight versus loose) and *interactivity* (complex versus linear) to analyse organisations. Health care is, however, nowhere to be seen in the early versions of Perrow's work. Snook (2000) has contributed the concept of *logic of action* with a potential axis of rule-based versus task-based actions. Unfortunately, models based on binary concepts like coupling, interactivity and logic of action distract us far too easily from the fact that complex systems are dynamic in their interactions with their surrounding environments.

Why has the nature of health care as a CAS attracted so little study and research? Perhaps the origin of this mystery can be found in part by concluding that health care is a 'very complex' CAS that has defied easy categorisation. Or perhaps the real difficulty arises from failing to recognise that a very different range of answers to the question (what sort of system is health care?) will be provided depending on whether we look at the system from the perspective of providers (including the full range from governments, to administrators, to clinicians and

1 This work offers a definition of CAS as a 'complex non-linear interactive system that has the ability to adapt to a changing environment' (p. 263).

2 A common and silly example of this 'exceptionalism' is seen in the comment 'Of course our outcomes are worse than the airline industry – you don't see 737 pilots flying planes full of frail elderly individuals with coronary artery disease and COPD, do you?'

other caregivers) or from the perspective of the recipients of the services.

The insight that we might look at health care from the perspective of the patients receiving that care will lead us to characterise the health care as a hybrid or heterogeneous CAS. At any given moment in time the patient's 'journey' will reflect the simultaneous activity of processes and sub-systems that are both loosely *and* tightly coupled as well as both linearly *and* complexly interactive, not to mention reflecting logics-of-action that are both task-based and rule-based. In other words, binary concepts may not be terribly useful to describe the dynamic nature of health care, when looked at from the patient's perspective. The case example below illustrates this heterogeneous nature of health care as a CAS.

Case Example

A 54 year-old man in a remote community was sent from a nursing station for the investigation of long-standing gastrointestinal dysfunction. A visiting specialist at a community hospital performed a gastroscopy and the biopsy reported several weeks later as showing a malignant tumour. The patient was referred to a major centre where surgery was performed.

During the wait for surgery, the patient consulted the nursing station again and was assessed. The results of the first referral were not available. The patient was referred to a different community hospital where another biopsy was undertaken, which was reported several weeks later (after the surgical intervention) as showing no malignancy along with chronic inflammation. The surgeon had no knowledge of the second biopsy. The surgical specimen also showed no malignancy.

The patient developed multiple disabling complications that can occur with such extensive surgery, even when performed perfectly, and was admitted to hospital 14 times in the next two years, always far from his home. None of the facilities (nursing station, two different community hospitals and major tertiary care centre) had any form of electronic record and no possibility of sharing information about the visits, procedures or pathology reports.

The investigation also revealed that 15 years earlier, a programme to train pathology technicians had been cancelled for fiscal and policy reasons. This led to a gradual prolongation of the time to report non-urgent pathology results from an average of one week before the cancellation to an average of four–six weeks at the time of this event. Clearly there had been a gradual acceptance of these delays as a form of 'new normal', reflecting the concept of normalisation of deviance.

The concept of health care as a particularly unusual type of CAS may help to explain the confusion around the various methods that are used to analyse adverse events. For some processes (typically those that are tightly coupled and linearly interactive), a simple linear approach may very well give an appropriate level of understanding of the event. For other processes or sub-system activities, the complex / complicated linear approach may suffice to provide a good understanding (and hopefully lead to effective learning) of what happened in a given case. The partial successes of these linear methods may lead investigators to ignore the fact that the processes and subsystems are in fact part of a complex adaptive socio-technical system and promote the application and use of linear methods in situations which do require a broader, holistic or systemic non-linear approach in order fully to make sense of what happened.

Application of the inappropriate investigation approach will (and does) lead to the generation of findings and recommendations that will not (and do not) address the real issues contributing to a given critical incident. The learning will be truncated, thus guaranteeing that the organisational change (adaptation) will be incomplete. Failure to appreciate the type of system in which the event occurred can easily lead to an inappropriate focus on individual components rather than on the relations between various elements of the system. At the same time, this can lead to a search for reliability rather than an understanding of and nurturing of the variability that is inherent in CAS. The issue of performance variability in the face of various environmental limitations is explored in detail in the FRAM (Hollnagel, 2012).

The application of a systemic non-linear approach to reviewing major events in health care will lead to a more robust understanding of the experience of a specific patient. This now brings us back to the purpose of this chapter – thinking about how to design workshops to educate system safety practitioners about systemic non-linear investigation approaches, taking into account the principles of complexity science and CAS theory.

How Do Complex Adaptive Systems Theory and Complexity Science Inform Incident Review Methods?

Over the past several decades, many seminal works have been written on the subject of complexity science and complex adaptive systems theory (Gleick, 1987; Stacey, 1992; Waldrop, 1992; Lorenz, 1993; Cilliers, 1998). While the authors write from different perspectives and focus on different types of systems, there is agreement about certain underlying principles and common characteristics of complex adaptive systems.

Cilliers (1998) has written very clearly about these principles and characteristics. Complex systems, generally speaking:

- are composed of a large number of elements that interact dynamically;
- are open living systems, with constant interaction with the surrounding environment, exchanging information and energy;
- exhibit primarily non-linear interactions and have many direct and indirect feedback loops;
- exhibit system properties and patterns of behaviour as a result of the dynamic interactions (internal and external) that propagate throughout the system;
- possess a memory that is typically distributed among the many components and elements.

When applied to complex socio-technical systems and organisations, Cilliers (1998) maintains that these characteristics are reflected in the following behaviours (all of which can be seen clearly in health care – see Kernick (2004) and Zimmerman (1998) for multiple examples):

- relationships are vital (interactions between components and semi-autonomous agents);
- context is crucial;
- history co-determines the nature of the complex organisation;
- unpredictability is a common feature of emergence;
- non-linearity leads to surprising outcomes – not always in proportion to the size or strength of a pattern or interaction;

- self-organisation tends to evolve such that the system is most sensitive to elements critical to its survival.

In order to make sense of events, it is important to understand the environment and context in which they evolve and occur. Any workshop that is intended to train safety practitioners to review events occurring in a CAS needs to demonstrate how the characteristics mentioned above are manifested and how they create conditions out of which will emerge the critical incident being investigated. Judging by the review of Lundberg, Rollenhagen and Hollnagel (2009), the eight examples of accident review methods in Sweden do not explore most of these issues nor do they equip investigators to understand the nature of complex socio-technical systems.

Designing an Effective Training Programme

Workshops in the field of conflict engagement and mediation are, for the most part, consciously designed so that the workshop structure and function actively embody and reflect the principles, techniques and values that are fundamental to effective performance of conflict management practitioners (Costantino and Merchant, 1996). This goes well beyond the principles of adult learning (Price, 2004), which in and of themselves, are important. Workshops designed to prepare safety practitioners to be effective event investigators, especially in the application of systemic non-linear methods, can replicate this approach.

The following are some of workshop design concepts (both in terms of substance and learning processes) that flow from an understanding of health care as a CAS:

1. Develop a Systemic / Holistic View of the Event

This should be a straightforward concept, but is often problematic in reality. We are interested in events that occur in a CAS and we should therefore provide content that will help safety practitioners understand the systemic context of the event. More to the point, the workshop material should be presented in a way that reflects CAS characteristics (for instance emergence, self-organisation). Instead, training workshops provide menus and checklists, reflecting a linear view of the world that is unlikely to be appropriate for CAS. The case example illustrates the value of a holistic approach in the analysis of this event.

2. Promote an Understanding of Non-linear Interactions and Linkages between Elements of a System

Price (2004) identifies several examples of non-linear learning methods, many of which can and should be incorporated into the training workshop approach. These include analysing case studies, the use of simulation and role-play, small group work, and problem-based learning techniques. These suggestions are inspired by the earlier work of Fraser and Greenhalgh (2001). It is important when integrating such techniques to talk openly about the non-linear nature of the learning experience.[3] As well, it is important to provide many examples, during the case studies, of CAS phenomena such as self-organisation, emergence and non-linearity (see the brief case example above). The workshop can go a long way to giving participants 'permission' to re-label (and indeed to 're-understand') phenomena according to some of the principles of complexity science, rather than always replicating linear mechanistic models of thought and analysis.

For instance, it is not uncommon to find examples, when reviewing critical incidents, of staff being obliged to ignore policies or procedures in order to solve problems that will also promote safety. Rather than labelling these with the rather pejorative term 'workarounds', we could just as easily describe these as examples of emergent patterns as a result of processes of self-organisation that occur in a CAS.

The case example reflects non-linearity clearly. It is extremely hard to imagine that the results of cancelling the training programme 15 years earlier could have been predicted or foreseen.

---

3 This refers to the unanticipated and unpredictable influence of other students and participants especially from sharing contextual elements of their own lived experiences. This often results in surprising leaps in learning.

3. Promote and Value the Narrative as a Central Way of Understanding What Happened (Letting the Stories Breathe[4])

Narratives are central to understanding events and phenomena in CAS. The importance of relational elements and interactions between various units, components, sub-systems, and the semi-autonomous agents that populate the CAS begin to surface and become obvious in the narrative. Attempting to structure the story (as often happens with paper-based or even web-based reporting forms consisting of many tick boxes) will lead to it being truncated and to the presentation of an artificial and incomplete view of the contextual and environmental conditions that existed at the time of the event in question. Klein (1998) provides valuable insights and suggestions about how to obtain the most revealing data and uncover the connections that are crucial to making sense of events. Frank (2010) illustrates, with many examples, exactly how stories can facilitate learning and stimulate the understanding of patterns in the listener or reader. For any given event being reviewed in a health care CAS, many stories will be 'constructed' (as opposed to a single 'true' account), reflecting the experience and social context of various players.

Some of our colleagues who may be uncomfortable with qualitative methodologies (or even worse, are simply ignorant of the validity of such methods) will dismiss stories and narratives as being merely 'anecdotes'. We should proceed cautiously and express sympathy in the face of such comments and demonstrate, through the structure and content of the training workshop, the power of the narrative.

4. Encourage Data Gathering (Quantitative and Qualitative) from a Wide Variety of Sources, Including Patients

This is a simple concept. Unfortunately, menu-driven or recipe-based linear investigation approaches have too often limited the areas that might be seen as useful sources of data. While this is true of many safety-critical domains, in health care, it is particularly manifested in the exclusion of the patient or family in the investigation process. The training workshop should bring

4 This is a slight modification of the title of a recent work by Frank (2010).

forward examples and case studies in which the observations or questions of patients and families were helpful in promoting a full understanding of the event in question. Finding such examples (assuming that you look for them) is not difficult and making the value-added nature of the input explicit for the training workshop participants is an obvious way of contributing to their understanding of the role of the patient / family as integral parts of the health care CAS.

5. Demonstrate the Application of Dialogic Data-gathering

This important concept underlies and supports the previous four suggestions about how to most effectively design a training programme for safety practitioners who will be reviewing critical incidents that occur in health care CAS. It is inspired by the work of Isaacs (1999), whose work *Dialogue: The Art of Thinking Together* outlines the elements of dialogue. Any workshop dealing with the investigation of events in CAS should be structured and should function in a fully dialogic fashion. This will facilitate the emergence of understanding about the operations of the CAS in question and will illustrate the richness of data that emerges from such an approach. Becoming skilled at leading dialogic discussions and inquiries is not an easy task and it would be wrong to create the impression that safety practitioners analysing adverse events will be fully comfortable after attending a workshop on systemic non-linear approaches. It will be important for the workshop faculty to be comfortable with the technique of dialogue. Demonstrating the application of the dialogic approach in the workshop will be an important step in moving the review / investigation processes away from linear menu-driven approaches that are less fruitful in CAS.

6. Demonstrate a Three-dimensional Dynamic Approach to Displaying Data

This is particularly challenging for health care personnel involved in reviewing critical incidents. Our world is one that seems to proceed in a strictly linear chronological fashion. Our records of treatment (hospital charts, consultation notes, operative and procedural notes) all reflect the linear chronological orientation that was both implicit and explicit in our initial training and subsequent inclusion in the health care field. Most investigation mapping depicts events as one-dimensional, proceeding in a linear fashion along an apparently 'flat' x-axis. Sometimes a second dimension is added, with the possibility of other elements combining with the main 'chronological highway' as they travel in from various positions on the y-axis. To truly capture the development of events in a CAS requires that we add a third dimension that we can label the z-axis and that can be seen as influences that move periodically and often stochastically upwards and outwards. This characterisation is developed by Dekker (2011a).

It is important for the training workshop to demonstrate the use of this kind of three-dimensional display in order for participants to more readily observe how the relational elements of the CAS at the time of the event emerge or become obvious. When applied to the case example, these relational links became obvious. Dekker (2006a) has observed that the way in which data is displayed can significantly influence how it is understood (the prime example being the distinction in the field of human factors between data *observability* and data *availability*). The training workshop provides the perfect setting to demonstrate this concept. A major advantage of the FRAM (Hollnagel, 2012) is the visual representation of functions in a manner that facilitates seeing the connections (called couplings) with other functions and thus the sites of potential resonance.

There are undoubtedly several other principles of complexity science and concepts derived from CAS theory that can be advantageously incorporated into training workshops for safety practitioners learning how to investigate major events in complex socio-technical adaptive systems. As experience is gained and comfort developed with this approach, additional concepts will be introduced.

Conclusion

This chapter has explored the question of designing workshops to train safety practitioners in the effective review or investigation of critical incidents occurring in health care CAS. An attempt has been made to understand how the basic principles of complexity science and CAS theory, when applied to health care (an example of a hybrid or heterogeneous CAS) will influence the design (in terms of both the content and the delivery processes) of such a workshop. The discussion has focused preferentially on systemic non-linear analytic approaches as being the most appropriate for making sense of events in CAS. Several suggestions have been advanced that pertain to this question. Other important concepts and principles will undoubtedly be added to supplement this analysis.

As noted at the beginning of the chapter, the retrospective review of 'things that go wrong' is firmly anchored in the perspective of Safety-I. The author is aware of evidence (as yet unpublished) that suggests that a systemic non-linear approach to such a Safety-I activity will yield useful results beyond a more robust understanding of a particular event or set of events in a CAS. One of these results will include gaining a fuller understanding of the functioning of a particular CAS, with particular emergence of insights into those elements that affect organisational resilience.

As yet, there is limited application of systemic non-linear approaches to prospective risk assessment of processes and events in health care CAS. Intuitively it makes sense that such an approach would also be useful if applied to prospective assessments and indeed, by facilitating a more fulsome and robust view of a given CAS, there is reason to think that the systemic non-linear approach will also bolster our ability to assess CAS-organisational resilience.

Chapter 17
Safety-II Thinking in Action: 'Just in Time' Information to Support Everyday Activities

Robyn Clay-Williams and Jeffrey Braithwaite

Introduction

There is a large body of literature on the use, benefits and particularly the challenges of information and communication technology (ICT) in health care (e.g., Bates and Gawande, 2003; Buntin et al., 2011), including many trials of information and decision support systems (e.g., Kaushal, Shojania and Bates, 2003; Roshanov et al., 2011; Gagnon et al., 2012). However, well integrated ICT systems, and good ways to use the data from these, are still in their infancy. While the data from integrated systems are utilised in other industries to improve safety and efficiency, the expectations of health care professionals of the benefits of integrated ICT systems are limited by their lack of experience with them. A clinician may think of a dashboard for clinical support (Mathe et al., 2009), for example, that aggregates disparate electronic patient records with decision-support components, as such a system. While these types of systems can provide timely access to patient data, they would only comprise one component of the 'just in time' information systems that we are proposing here.

Over the last decade, health care has looked to high safety industries such as aviation for ideas on how to improve care in risky environments, including exploiting ICT. Many parts of health care are exposed to, and require, high variability. It is therefore misguided to transfer solutions that have been designed for – and work well in – highly regular and regulated environments. In any case, take-up of ICT has been variable, and degrees of risk in different disciplines of medicine are furthermore uneven. The challenges are considerable, so we need to tease out the problems facing us.

Risk and Resilience

Traditional approaches to safety involve attempting to minimise the number of things that go wrong. This thinking, which is known as Safety-I, is grounded in the idea that things that go wrong are caused by different processes to things that go right. Safety-I thinking can lead to effective solutions in industries where processes are linear and modes of failures are repetitive or predictable. Complex adaptive systems, however – such as health care – are intractable. Adding Safety-I solutions such as barriers or layers of defence risks making it more so. Things that go wrong are often not predictable in time, place or character, and there is greater leverage to be achieved by looking at what goes right. This type of thinking, which is termed Safety-II, accepts that the processes are the same regardless of whether the outcome is positive or negative, and involves a more proactive approach to error management. A detailed description of Safety-I and Safety-II thinking can be found in Chapter 1.

If we look at risk through a Safety-I conceptual model, applied to a variety of industries, we find that anaesthetics and blood transfusion fall into a similar risk category to commercial aviation and railways. However, when we look at medicine overall, the likelihood of encountering adverse events can be far higher (Amalberti et al., 2005). It is not just the larger number of adverse events in health care, however, but the poor predictability of the type of events or the timing of occurrence that makes Safety-I thinking problematic.

It is becoming increasingly evident that industry safety management methods promoting high reliability, such as standardisation and regulatory supervision, are less applicable in health care due to the variability, complexity and need for flexibility in diagnosing and treating patients. In high reliability industries, if the equipment or workplace processes are wearing out, then they are replaced so that failures remain unlikely. Yet in health care, the machine equivalent is the technology, processes and clinical journey we put patients through, which seem by nature almost always to be out of date or in a poor state of repair, mainly due to resource pressures. If we inserted regulatory or bureaucratic barriers to every potential failure as in aviation, people might legitimately worry that we would run out of money to pay for it all, or that health care would grind to a halt.

So, how do we encourage improvements as indicated by Safety-II thinking, while retaining our ability to deal flexibly with complexity and variability? The answer seems to lie in managing system resilience, and providing real-time data is core to this. We have to do some systems thinking to appreciate this point. Resilience is 'the intrinsic ability of a system to adjust its functioning prior to, during, or following changes and disturbances, so that it can sustain required operations under both expected and unexpected conditions' (Hollnagel, 2011b).

An apparent paradox of resilience is that it is likely to be higher in organisations where risk is greater. It is apparent, because resilience is less needed, if at all, for highly regulated and ordered activities. The more practice people get doing work or resolving crises, the better they become at it. This is well known across medicine: amongst the classic instances are triage capabilities in war-torn environments, and surgeons with high volumes becoming more skilled than their less busy, or less specialised, counterparts.

Clinicians as individuals are relatively autonomous and build personal resilience because they become experienced at solving complex, unique and time-critical problems with incomplete information. There is a feeling of resignation in some circles that safety in health care cannot be improved without sacrificing this hard-won autonomy and natural resilience because it will mean more bureaucracy and regulation. For many clinicians this is too high a price to pay (Braithwaite and Clay-Williams, 2012).

Military Aviation as an Exemplar

However, if we look to another industry such as military aviation, which has different properties from the commercial aviation model normally applied to health care, we can see that flexibility, resilience and safety are not mutually exclusive concepts. In peacetime, military aviation operates in a regulatory safety environment comparable to commercial aviation. However, in time of war or disaster relief operations, military aviation requires a similar flexibility and resilience to health care. It does things fast, under the pressure of emergent complexity, with information made available very close to the time decisions are made. Military aviation also operates under conditions of uncertainty, which may be as important as conditions of time pressure. While military training incorporates lessons in how to deal with contingency, performance in the field depends to an extent on innovation and improvisation based on circumstances as they arise. Planning for something that is unknown or unpredictable is not possible, so we must rely on the ability to adjust performance in real time. In the last two decades, US military aviation has perhaps surprisingly managed to do this while retaining overall operational safety levels comparable to those in anaesthetics (Wiegmann and Shappell, 1999; O'Connor et al., 2012; Gibb and Olson, 2008). Although priorities and values change, the requirements to achieve mission objectives and to protect high value assets – such as aircraft, and key, well-trained people – remain. In military aviation, it is recognised that the requirements of war are incompatible with peacetime levels of control. Therefore appropriate boundaries or rules of engagement are set and personnel are trained to be resilient when operating at, or near, these boundaries.

Like military aviation in wartime, health care is a dynamic system subject to continuous production pressures and with changing and often uncontrollable boundaries. Figure 17.1 (Cook and Rasmussen, 2005) depicts a typical operating envelope of a health care system, and shows the elements that can put pressure on the boundaries.

Pressures from management and increased patient demands shrink the space for safe operation, and squeeze the typical operating point towards the boundary of acceptable safe performance. This boundary has a margin for error which itself can vary depending on prevailing conditions. Cook and Rasmussen have shown that '... precise knowledge of the dynamics and

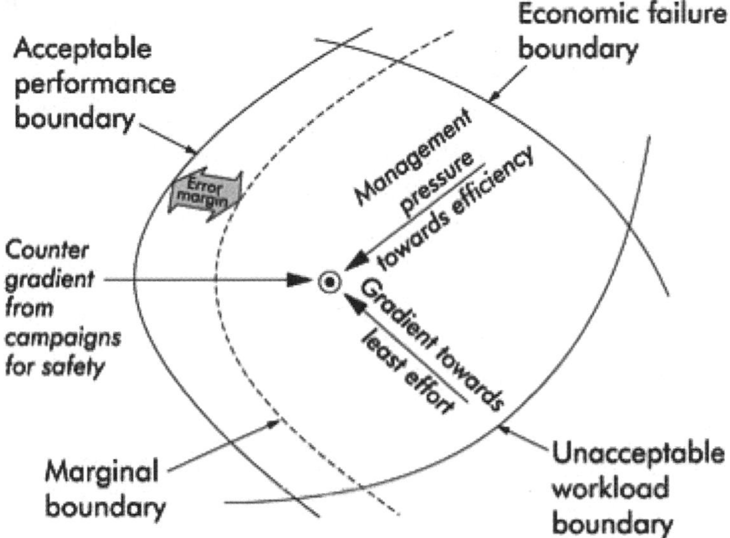

Figure 17.1 System operating point

Source: Reproduced from Cook, R.I. and Rasmussen, J. (2005). 'Going solid': A model of system dynamics and consequences for patient safety. Quality and Safety in Health Care, *14(2), 131. With permission from BMJ Publishing Group Ltd.*

location of the current operating point and boundary locations is a necessary component of a safety culture' (Cook and Rasmussen, 2005: 133). This is complicated in health care, as the boundaries in real life are frequently not visible, and they can change rapidly as circumstances vary. Currently, the only way of determining where the boundary of safe operations lies for any given situation is by pushing the envelope until there are signs that safety has been breached. This is hardly an acceptable state of affairs.

The Need for 'Just in Time' Information

Resilience engineering shows us that there are alternate ways of improving safety. Resilience engineering is not just about controlling risk, but 'attaining better control of the control of risk' (Dekker, 2006b: 82). Consequences of adjustments need to be made inferable before actions are taken, so that we can identify any potentially harmful outcomes. For this we need information, but not the way we currently get it, and even not the way we are currently planning to get it with new ICT systems. What we really need is not so much information about where the system is now, but rather, where it's going to be 15 minutes from now. So, in similar ways to military aviation, health care needs information in real time, or close to real time. 'Just in time' information is defined as information that is available in a timeframe where it is relevant to make critical decisions for patient care. When a system departs from the norm, it is easier to recover if action is taken early, when the departure is only small. 'Just in time' information allows deviations to be identified earlier and corrective action taken. Put in health care terms, busy clinicians making critical decisions would have relevant data available at their fingertips. Instead, most information is presently in inaccessible forms, not immediately available at the point the decision is made, or captured in reports that appear weeks or months too late.

In health care today patient information is increasingly stored in multiple computer systems that clinical professionals use when delivering patient care. There are many of these idiosyncratic computer systems as a result of every clinical entity having (or wanting) their own information system that meets their needs – and as a result of effective sales talk (Goldfinch, 2007). Theoretically at least, the resultant data could be aggregated into user-friendly configurations, allowing these data to be collated and displayed in a coherent, meaningful way, in a format matched to the workflow requirements of the user, available 'just in time'. Leveson advocates the importance of making autonomous decisions 'in the context of system level information and from a total systems perspective in order to be effective in reducing accidents' (Leveson et al., 2009: 237).

Yet we are swamped with oceans of data – what has been called the data deluge (Szalay and Gray, 2006). Getting a 'total' systems perspective, or a 'total' patient view, is therefore problematic. Many attempts have been made to collect this information in an aggregated view but in many cases the information is organised for administrative, quality, or research purposes in disconnected systems, and is primarily retrospective. The information needs to be salient, and it needs to be available when it is required to support delivery of patient care. Even the new ICT systems proposed for health care (Bates and Gawande, 2003; Buntin et al., 2011; Kaushal, Shojania and Bates, 2003; Gagnon et al., 2012;

Goldfinch, 2007) fall short for the most part in imagining they can address 'just in time' requirements.

Because health care is complex and continually evolving, there is often a difference between work-as-imagined and work-as-done. While management may expect clinicians to follow prescribed rules and procedures to the letter, in reality workarounds are often necessary to meet time and production targets (Gabbay and May, 2004). Sometimes the procedures are outdated, not relevant, conflicting with other goals, or impracticable, and departures are required in order to provide the best treatment for the patient. Organisations are brittle where there is a disconnect between how management believe work is done, and how tasks are actually accomplished at the 'coalface' (Dekker, 2011a). This is analogous to Argyris's 'theory espoused' versus 'theory in use' (Argyris, 2010): members of an organisation believe that they are acting in a particular way, usually that aligned with the organisation's vision, mission and values. In reality, however – as a result of production and social pressures – they are behaving quite differently. And managers may harbour still another set of beliefs about how members are behaving. Availability of timely and accurate information may help focus collective efforts, and build system resilience.

Getting the Information We Need

We need to do a thought experiment about this for a moment: what if people could get just the information they wanted and only when they need it? How is it possible to determine ahead of time which information people want (or need) and when? It may be possible if work-as-done closely corresponds to work-as-imagined, but that in turn implies compliance and Safety-I thinking. If the situation is not well structured – and in health care it often is not – then the information needs to be available on demand and in a flexible format to meet the situational needs of the clinician.

Although there is no simple solution to this dilemma, and although there are many issues to resolve, this may not be the pipe dream many people think. Real-time data are starting to become available to decision makers in other industries. Central banks are beginning to use real-time data to construct 'nowcasts' of economic markers such as GDP and inflation, although demonstrated success is still very limited (Giannone, Reichlin and Small, 2008). The military is also starting to use synthesised real-time data to make key tactical decisions during battles (Schmidt, Corsaro and van't Hag, 2008). It is now possible to process and display real-time data in health care: patterns can be identified in electronic health care data distributed over multiple systems, allowing clinicians access to data in formats that facilitate improvement in the delivery of care (Plaisant et al., 2008). Recently, paediatricians at a US hospital were able to collate electronic medical record (EMR) data, where no other evidence sources were available, to decide whether anticoagulation was the safest treatment for a 13-year-old patient with systemic lupus erythematosus (SLE) (Frankovich, Longhurst and Sutherland, 2011). Although this took several hours, it allowed treatment to be based on evidence (rather than trial and error) and was therefore in a suitable time frame to meet the needs of the clinicians and the patient. Unlike for the cost of bureaucratic systems or rigid ICT systems being implemented in many countries now, this might be worth paying for.

Yet examples in health care are few and far between. Improvements in efficiency, accelerating demands and scarce resources mean that health care systems of today are operating close to or at capacity. There are few buffers. The tightly coupled nature of delivery systems means that safety properties of medical practice can change rapidly, and propagate through the organisation. Problems in one area of the hospital may result from activities in another area that may be only peripherally related (Rasmussen, 1997). Change the procedures in theatres or pathology, for instance, and doctors down the line in emergency, outpatients or general practice are affected. Hospitals crippled by bed-block are another case in point. A critical component in improving performance could be access to timely information.

Conclusion

Safe decisions are easier to make if the future is less uncertain. Clinicians and health care managers need real-time information in order to provide a window into potential paths and to reduce the uncertainty or ameliorate it. Argyris (1999) states that this is one of the core characteristics of a learning organisation. Predictive information would enhance the ability to anticipate, which is one of the central themes in resilience engineering and Safety-II thinking. Surely, progress with 'just in time' information systems, on which to make the necessary complex and time-critical decisions needed to treat patients effectively, is key to strengthening safety at the boundaries? And just as surely, ought we to learn from nowcasting in banking, military aviation in wartime, and the occasional example drawn from health care, to tackle the 'just in time' problem, with the golden opportunity to promote resilience?

Chapter 18
Mrs Jones Can't Breathe: Can a Resilience Framework Help?

Patricia H. Strachan

Introduction

Resilience in health care is most often discussed in relation to disasters or emergency conditions under which the system becomes stressed in dramatic ways that affect a number of people at a time. This would include patients, practitioners and the community or health system at large who experience a large-scale accident or epidemic (Bhamra, Dani and Burnard, 2011). While it is tempting and necessary to be drawn to such situations, it is also important that resilience is examined within the everyday world of an organisation and in the context of health care, in relation to the individuals who rely on such organisations to receive care. One such significant group of individuals is those who suffer from a progressive, chronic, life-limiting illness such as heart failure (HF).

This chapter is intended to promote discussion about the application of a resilience framework to the challenge of providing comprehensive, safe and compassionate care to patients with advanced HF. The following text will:

- outline the health context (specifically, advanced HF) from which resilience will be examined and consider the relationship between *individual* resilience and *system* or *organisational* resilience;

- apply the four basic abilities of a resilient organisation to the context of advanced HF care;
- propose questions and approaches to be considered about how the potential for a resilience framework could promote important, safe and compassionate patient-centered care for those who live with advanced HF and other progressive, chronic life-limiting illness.

Resilience in Progressive, Life-limiting Chronic Illness: The Case for Heart Failure

Heart failure (HF) is an example of a progressive, chronic, life-limiting illness that most commonly affects older adults. It is a complex, chronic syndrome in which the heart has a decreased ability to meet metabolic demands, in the advanced stages causing suffering and marked decreases in quality of life due to fatigue, shortness of breath, depression and activity restrictions. Altered cognitive function, nausea, abdominal distention and discomfort are typical as the condition advances to an end-stage (Beattie and Goodlin, 2008).

HF is a major cause of morbidity and mortality in developed countries; better therapies and an ageing population contribute to predictions that numbers affected will increase (Ko et al., 2008). HF is one of the most common reasons for hospitalisation of older adults; it has a high readmission rate and is associated with escalating economic costs (Chun et al., 2012). Together these issues underscore the importance this illness has for individual patients, the health care system and society at large.

Patients with advanced HF commonly experience variations of an undulating and unpredictable illness trajectory punctuated by potentially life-threatening exacerbations from which they are routinely saved by (individuals within) the emergency health care system, hospitalised for a time and return home (Beattie and Goodlin, 2008). For this reason, patients are often viewed by themselves, their families and those in the health care system as 'resilient' individuals; a label many patients wear proudly. In fact, it is the patient's ability to bounce back from the brink of death when experiencing acute pulmonary oedema, and the acute care (sub)system's consistent ability to assist patients to do this, that has led to a resilience paradox. Although individual and sub-system responses to acute exacerbations create the appearance of resilience, these responses (as measured by outcomes such as resuscitation time, length of stay, mortality) are evaluated (if at all) in isolation with limited linkage to the broader context that has influenced the patient's deterioration and need for emergent care. Thus, when system elements of anticipating, monitoring, responding and learning focus only on the acute episode, many, including the patient, would conclude that the health care system is functioning well, when it is actually inadequate and the sub-systems are not interacting optimally. Instead, a truly resilient HF care system would be reflected in non-events (such as reduced need for emergency care).

It is postulated that failure to consider and explore the inter-relationships between the individual and the organisation may have a negative impact on the potential for the complex health care system to develop broader organisational resilience that would better serve patients. Of increasing concern is that the confluence of individual and organisational resilience has created conditions in which important and patient-centred communication about prognosis, goals of care, advance care planning and the possibility of palliative care have been muted for patients with advanced HF. Patients live with the consequences of this; unrelieved and / or poorly managed symptoms, suboptimal death experiences and significant stress, and care-giver burden on their families (Beattie and Goodlin, 2008; Kaasalainen et al., 2011). Meanwhile, health care systems grapple with the economic and human costs of responding to the recurring crises in an ever-increasing population of potential users.

Although resilience is often referred to as a valued characteristic for a patient, family or community, it has seldom been the specific focus *per se* of discussions about chronic illness in relation to system issues. While many reports and research publications call for a better system of care to serve patients with conditions such as HF, making that happen remains a formidable challenge.

Mrs Jones: One of the Many Faces of Advanced Heart Failure

There are many characteristics shared by those who live with advanced HF. They tend to be older adults, have co-morbidities, use polypharmacy, require assistance to access care and due to human resource challenges, may not be under the care of a HF cardiologist or specialty clinic (Heckman et al., 2007). Mrs Jones is an amalgam of the thousands of individuals with advanced HF in Canada. She is 78, has had two previous heart attacks, one of which required angioplasty and the stenting of three coronary vessels. She has a pacemaker. She is on several medications, is moderately hypertensive, and also suffers from Type II diabetes mellitus. She lives at a long-term care facility (LTC). Her general practitioner visits once a month. Every three months, her daughter transports her to the heart failure clinic at a tertiary care hospital where a cardiologist adjusts her medications. Her pacemaker function is also monitored by the arrhythmia service in the same hospital every six months.

Over the past week, she has felt unwell and has been less active, sometimes taking her meals in her room. She was not sleeping well, waking frequently at night. On the night in question she became acutely short of breath and diaphoretic. This information was transmitted to the nurse supervisor, who called an ambulance to transport Mrs Jones to a community hospital ten minutes away. She was quickly placed in the resuscitation area in the emergency department (ED). An emergency physician determined that she was in pulmonary oedema (a common, acute and life-threatening complication of HF) and instituted prompt treatment. Over the next hour her vital signs stabilised and her oxygen saturation improved. Because of her history of previous cardiac problems (and particularly because of her two visits to this ED in the past year for virtually identical presentations), she was admitted for two days. Upon discharge home to a LTC facility, a revised list of prescribed medications was sent, with no other instructions for changes in everyday care.

Patients like Mrs Jones are likely to die sometime in the next year (Hutt et al., 2011). She is not likely to have any understanding of the natural progression of her illness nor have an advance care plan to guide decisions about goals of care (Strachan et al., 2009). She will suffer significantly due to the system failure to anticipate her needs as she moves along the illness trajectory and efforts to minimise her suffering will focus on the increasingly frequent acute episodes.

Looking for Resilience in the Context of Care

Drawing from the definition of organisational resilience according to Hollnagel (2011b), a resilient HF care system must be able to adjust its function in anticipation of and in response to the individually unpredictable care needs of those who live with advanced HF, in a way that maintains the integrity of the system as a whole, remaining open and able to satisfactorily respond to the needs of others who require care at any time. To assess its resilience, we might ask which system are we looking at or perhaps from whose point of view the resilience is being examined. For instance, the ED physicians and nurses who quickly resuscitated Mrs Jones think of the ED as a system unto itself. This narrow conception of the care system typifies what has been termed a siloed approach to health care that is common within practice environments. Other sub-systems such as the heart failure clinic and the LTC home have tended to engage in similar internally focused examinations and, to a much lesser degree, the relationships between the sub-systems.

Mrs Jones (when her cognitive functioning allows her to think about the question) and her family perceive the system of care to include the community hospital ED, the ambulance service, the family physician, the cardiologist at the HF clinic, the advanced practice nurse at the pacemaker clinic at the tertiary care centre, and the LTC home (and their employees). This expanded view of the system fits with the organisational model of care that is most often developed and endorsed at a planning and policy level of the health care system. Evidently, the mental model by which the system (or sub-system) is viewed, planned for, lived in and evaluated, is of critical importance to understanding its resilience. The following analysis will examine these models using the attributes of organisational resilience – anticipating, responding, monitoring and learning (Hollnagel, 2011b: xxxvii).

Evaluating the Resilience Attributes

Anticipating

The many sub-systems involved with and relevant to the care of patients with chronic conditions recognise and anticipate the potential for patients like Mrs Jones to require emergent care. For those in the emergency care system, this is routinely anticipated; emergency response and ED staff maintain competence by staying current with and establishing local protocols derived from the extensive evidence-based HF guidelines that exist. There are concerns about the revolving door phenomenon experienced by a growing number of patients like Mrs Jones who are living with chronic, progressive life-limiting illness. Re-hospitalisations and recurrent ED visits are associated with poor prognosis and increased mortality rates (Hutt et al., 2011; Chun et al., 2012). In the future, more chronically ill patients who survive acute exacerbations will require admission to hospital. When they eventually deteriorate and can no longer function independently, greater demand will be placed on the under-resourced chronic care system.

Ironically, despite the numbers of patients suffering from HF, HF-specific care driven by HF guidelines is rare in LTC sub-systems (Heckman et al., 2007; Marcella et al., 2012). A recent large-scale investigation in Ontario, Canada, reported that LTC facilities were often staffed by unregulated care providers and supervised by a skeleton crew of nurses, some with limited understanding of HF (Marcella et al., 2012). LTC settings are challenged in their capacity to provide more than summoning an ambulance when patients suddenly decompensate. Some unique programs have begun to have emergency HF-specific medication kits in LTC settings, but this remains a rarity.

Anticipation of emergency and ongoing chronic care for HF is variable at other system levels. Mrs Jones and her family have had no concrete discussions about the possibility of her death; no advanced care planning has been done to determine the limits of goals of care, including resuscitation and all it may entail. This is consistent with findings about seriously ill patients hospitalised with HF (Strachan et al., 2009) and other chronic life-limiting illnesses (Heyland et al., 2006) across Canada, the majority of whom had many unmet needs for information, communication and support related to end-of-life care and planning. Further, although HF guidelines now advocate for palliative and end-of-life care for patients with HF (Goodlin et al., 2004; Jaarsma et al., 2009; McKelvie et al., 2011), many practitioners are uncomfortable with questions related to end-of-life decision making and there are common concerns amongst many practitioners about if and when palliative care is relevant for patients with HF, although in-roads are slowly being made in this regard (LeMond and Allen, 2011).

Responding

The successful response to Mrs Jones's acute distress reflects that although LTC staff have limited knowledge and expertise with HF (Marcella et al., 2012), they did recognise the urgent situation and the emergency sub-system reacted well to meet her immediate physiological needs. She survived the immediate threat to life. But what about her ongoing heart health? We can predict that almost 50 per cent of similar patients will die within a year (Hutt et al., 2011); those who survive longer will suffer significantly as the HF worsens (Beattie and Goodlin, 2008). Lack of co-ordination between sub-systems makes the sharing of information problematic (Pratt Hopp et al., 2010). The family doctor may only learn of this acute episode at the time of the next monthly visit to the LTC. There is no mechanism by which the cardiologist or the pacemaker clinic will be certain to learn of this episode. In addition to the new medication list, LTC personnel are most likely to receive (if at all and after some time), only a brief summary of the hospital course (Marcella et al., 2012). LTC residents who suffer from advanced HF do not currently receive the care as advocated by the consensus-driven HF guidelines (Heckman, 2007, Low et al., 2011).

Reactive rather than proactive HF management tends to be the norm; this occurs even when patients are managed at home, where they engage in self-care. Although self-care has been identified as the cornerstone of HF management, there has been limited success in its implementation (Riegel et al., 2009). It is not uncommon that small HF-related changes that develop in patients over a few days to weeks may be noticed but not acted upon, until the patient is in an acute and often life-threatening crisis that requires emergent care.

Monitoring

At the level of the individual patient, consistent and useful monitoring of day-to-day fluctuations in physiologic status that could detect and manage problems before an acute exacerbation occurs would potentially benefit the patient and the health care system by decreasing the need for emergent care and related suffering. Recent efforts to implement daily–weekly weight monitoring for HF patients in LTC have proven to be a difficult, if not impossible, intervention due to the complexities of the sub-system of LTC care. Small weight increases (i.e., 1–2.5 kg) beginning a week prior to hospitalisation reflect decreasing cardiac muscle function resulting in fluid accumulation and are known to be early indicators of impending HF-related decline (Chaudry et al., 2007). They are often amenable to early intervention that would prevent hospitalisation, yet this knowledge fails to be monitored and subsequently used effectively in the LTC system.

In home settings, such monitoring depends on the consistency with which patients engage with HF self-care; this may be shared with or delegated to a family or LTC caregiver. HF self-care has received little rigorous attention from the medical community other than a recognition it is lacking. For instance, adherence to HF medications has been documented as ranging between 2 and 90 per cent (Riegel et al., 2009), reflecting that the prescription of medication alone is an insufficient indicator of care. Despite what is increasingly recognised about the importance of family caregivers to a patient's HF self-care and their use of the health care system, the caregiver contribution, needs and consequent sequelae (known as caregiver burden) have been virtually ignored and not measured as an outcome. HF self-care maybe monitored by clinicians, although no standardised tool for that currently exists; subsequently its utility as an indicator of wellness or impending decompensation has yet to be determined. Research to understand these care complexities is challenging to undertake in this population, leaving us with considerable knowledge gaps (Fitzsimons and Strachan, 2012); HF research has largely focused on outcomes in healthier HF subjects related to high tech interventions such as medications, medical devices and invasive procedures that are more amenable to clinical trials.

Learning

In the case of Mrs Jones, both the process and outcome of care were apparently positive, reinforcing the protocols in place for emergent care of a patient in fulminant pulmonary oedema. Because of this, it is likely that no further analysis would be routinely undertaken and no formalised learning would be sought out nor engaged in by any part of the system (LTC, emergency responders, ED). Since most of the other stakeholders did not receive information about the acute episode, it is challenging for them to learn, unless they have set up a proactive system to keep in touch with Mrs Jones, her family and her immediate care providers in LTC. In a small percentage of cases, this may be occurring but it is likely that, in the absence of a critical incident, any learning is focused on management of Mrs Jones's acute episode. At an ED sub-system level, we may learn about how quickly we can turn a patient's condition around, how quickly we can transfer them out of the department (the ED or in-patient unit) or institution and perhaps at some level, what interventional approach works best. But what do we learn about keeping them out of hospital, about reducing suffering for them and their family caregiver, about the needs of the LTC setting or adapting the HF guidelines so that they can work in LTC – all of which could offer Mrs Jones an opportunity to stay out of hospital and if relevant, to live well until the point of death, to die with dignity and without suffering?

In fact, we have learned very little. There is a paucity of integrated knowledge from across the system of HF care, including how the local operators (clinicians) and the institutional culture in which they work can best serve these patients. This imperative to learn about the relationships amongst those in the system as a whole and local components or agents in the subsystem (Pariès, 2011: 7) is one which continues to challenge us.

Discussion: How Resilient is the System of Care for Persons with Advanced Heart Failure?

The assessment of resilience based on the four identified attributes provides a general overview of some of the contextual challenges of caring for patients who require care from more than one sub-system within the larger health care system. It also raises many questions about both the system (and sub-systems) of HF care and how and what we could choose to learn that could better serve patients. The resilient (or perhaps pseudo-resilient) nature of individual patients with advanced HF may lead one to believe the system is more resilient than it actually is. In other words, when patients get better and bounce back from adversity, we tend to assume the system has been working efficiently and that care processes have unfolded as they should to lead to these improvements. Particularly when marginalised, vulnerable patients such as Mrs Jones survive and it appears we have 'saved' them from death, there may be little impetus to examine and learn about the degree of system resilience.

We have little understanding about situations in which patients with advanced HF are successfully managed in sub-systems of care (for instance, primary health care settings, community, LTC) and do not require hospital-based acute or emergency care. Arguably, a truly resilient system of HF care would be one in which there would be coordinated and integrated relationships between clinicians, patients and caregivers across sub-systems effectively to avoid and / or manage emergency situations outside the acute care setting. Examination of these care contexts is required for us truly to understand the distinction between apparent and real resilience at the individual and organisational level.

At a system level, many indicators that could be monitored to assess the integrity of the cardiac care system have been proposed but their uptake requires commitment at all levels of the health care system with investment of fiscal and human infrastructure to be successful (Boyd and Murray, 2010; Howlett et al., 2010). New and contextually relevant indicators are necessary for resilience to be adequately assessed in situations such as the one presented. It is paramount this would include items in addition to those relating to crisis (such as hospitalisation or death), and that are part of the sometimes mundane existence of those who require chronic (HF) care. This would include measurement of the quantity and quality of advance care planning, transitional care between sub-systems, self-care and its support, symptom management (such as weighing patients to assess fluid retention), timely palliative care provision, caregiver contribution and relationships between all stakeholders. Focusing investigations on the features and processes of LTC settings instead of medications, devices and procedures (Hutt et al., 2011) and the inter-relationships between individual and health care sub-systems offers necessary possibilities for increasing system resilience and improving the experience for patients living with HF (Ryder et al., 2011; Newhouse et al., 2012).

Conclusion

Care provision and decisions about the depth and breadth of system boundaries to which resilience thinking is applied are inherently moral activities. A resilience framework that offers a new lens by which care of patients with chronic illness like advanced HF can be analysed, is necessary if we are to create health care systems that are 'morally habitable places' (Austin, 2007: 86) for all stakeholders. Patients living with progressive life-limiting chronic illness, require, seek and experience care in many and various sub-systems that make up what is referred to as the health care system. Thus, if we are to analyse, recognise and facilitate resilience, we must identify and understand the system or sub-system involved. For these patients to experience safe, compassionate and excellent gold-standard care, the relationships between these sub-systems are also critical: all aspects of the system must work well for these patients and their families.

Epilogue: How to Make Health Care Resilient

Erik Hollnagel, Jeffrey Braithwaite and Robert L. Wears

The difference between theory and practice is larger in practice than in theory.

Introduction

Throughout this book the chapters have argued for the need to go beyond a Safety-I perspective and adopt a Safety-II perspective. Sheps and Cardiff (Chapter 5), Wears and Vincent (Chapter 11), Chuang (Chapter 14), Hollnagel (Chapter 1) and Amalberti (Chapter 3) in particular tender coherent arguments about, and support for, this advice. This is, however, not meant as an exclusive proposition where a focus on why things go wrong is *replaced* by a focus on why things go right, but rather as an inclusive proposition where a Safety-II perspective complements a Safety-I perspective. A Safety-I perspective is still needed because it is important to pay attention to that which goes wrong and to learn lessons from the accreted knowledge. But we also need a Safety-II perspective, both to avoid being constrained by the traditional preoccupation with failures, and to widen the understanding of why things sometimes go wrong but mostly do not. If there are gold nuggets in learning from Safety-I activities, there are rich golden seams to be mined in understanding the myriad of everyday activities that make care succeed. In Chapter 2, Cook traces the development of some key aspects of this logic.

The chapters have also illustrated the consequences of adopting a Safety-II perspective by way of realistic examples: Pariès, Lot, Rome and Tassaux (Chapter 7) provide an in-depth review of an ICU, Nyssen and Blavier (Chapter 8) consider robotic surgery, and Fairbanks, Perry, Bond and Wears (Chapter 13) illuminate the complexities we face by looking at the contrasting cases of failure in a resilient system and success in a brittle system. The question is therefore not *whether* we should try to make health care resilient, but *what* we should do to turn the principles of Safety-II into practices. Taking the collected advice of all the chapters, where and how should we begin to make care resilient? What are the practical steps needed to build a resilient health care system?

Work-as-Imagined and Work-as-Done

Everyone knows that they can only do their work by continually adjusting what they do to the conditions. Because performance adjustments are always necessary, work-as-done (WAD) is always different from work-as-imagined (WAI). This is so both at the sharp end, across the clinical 'coalface', and at the blunt end, amongst the management layers. The two terms were introduced to explain how proximal or sharp-end factors (acting here and now) in combination with distal or blunt-end factors (acting there and then) could lead to accidents (Reason, 1993; Hollnagel, 2004). Because the focus was on adverse events, nearly all attention was given to what people did at the sharp end, and this focus has remained.

It is unfortunate that whereas accidents are experienced by people at the actual sharp end, it is people at the blunt end who are responsible for preventing them. Because of the focus on the sharp end, everybody noticed the performance variability that took place there and happily used that as an explanation for incidents and adverse events (conveniently relabelled 'human error' or some such). Yet few noticed that performance at the blunt end was at least as variable and relied at least as much on performance adjustments as at the sharp end (cf. Hollnagel, 2004). People at the sharp end accept that WAD is, and must be, different from WAI. For them, it is no surprise that descriptions based on WAI cannot be used in practice and that actual work is different from prescribed work. People at the blunt end, however, do not see this as easily and therefore believe there should be no distinction between WAI and WAD, using any difference between them to explain why things went wrong. Since managers rarely look at how they do their own work, spending their time 'looking down' rather than 'looking within', they can conveniently use this belief to guide their understanding of why adverse events happen and of how safety should be managed.

Unlike Safety-I, Safety-II considers WAD at the sharp end and the blunt end on equal terms, and recognises that performance adjustments are required in both cases. Safety-II acknowledges that WAI and WAD are different, but draws the conclusion that one must study WAD to understand why.

The Naivety Trap

To make health care resilient, we must avoid the common belief that specific problems have specific solutions that can be applied without having to consider whether there are other consequences than the intended and desired ones. This belief is at best naïve and at worst harmful. In reality, health care cannot be made resilient by solving the problems one by one, in a step-by-step fashion. It requires a systemic approach. Health care is not a simple, linear mechanism but a complex adaptive system (CAS) – or even an autopoietic system. Robson (Chapter 16) and Braithwaite, Clay-Williams, Nugus and Plumb (Chapter 6) make this point, and tease out some of the main CAS characteristics of health care. Crucially, one cannot change one thing, one procedure, one task, in isolation or by itself. Any specific solution to a problem will have effects that are potentially widespread and in most cases unimagined – though not necessarily unimaginable. This requires multiple perspectives, and is the reason why it is necessary to have patients involved and to encourage them to be active agents both in their care and systems changes – the case for which is articulated by Gorini, Mazzocco and Pravettoni (Chapter 15).

Changes, of course, sometimes have to be made to address a concrete problem. But this should not be done without first having thought through the rest, trying as far as possible to anticipate what impact a proposed change will have on the rest of the system. This must include estimates of when the effects of the change have become established, so that a new change is not introduced before the previous one has had its effect – and the system has reached a reasonably steady state. A proper systemic approach must include an assessment of the consequences of changes before they are made – including defining measures, estimating delays and considering the effects on other parts of the system. It is important to avoid what Merton (1936) called the 'imperious immediacy of interest', which means that a dominant interest in immediate (or primary) results leads to a disregard of side effects.

Embedding and Supporting RHC

In resilience engineering, resilience is not so much a quality that a system *has* as a characteristic of how it functions, i.e., what it *does*. Several chapters have used – either explicitly or implicitly – the general idea that a system, in order to be resilient, must be able to respond, monitor, learn, and anticipate.

It is practically impossible to specify precisely what resilient performance will look like, and therefore also directly to engineer it. The adjustments that people make – the trade-offs and 'sacrifices' – are the results of individual or collective decision making rather than an engineered feature. This has been described either as 'muddling through' (Lindblom, 1959), meaning that decisions are made through successive limited comparisons, or as satisficing – that is, finding a solution that works, under conditions of bounded rationality (Simon, 1947; 1956). The choices are made during system transients with unpredictable (and often inadequate) resources and equally unpredictable (and often excessive) demands. This situation dependence makes it practically impossible to micro-manage performance adjustments. Performance, successes and failures alike, requires the ability to adjust in the given situation in a measured, thoughtful way that characterises smooth adaptation to the system's challenges. Attempting to engineer that would remove the genuinely needed spontaneity. Instead, the ability to make the right adjustments can and should be facilitated and supported, and perhaps even prepared.

The adjustments have sometimes been characterised as goal sacrifices but are actually a mixture of exchanging goals and of substituting means. Exchanging goals means that some objectives are abandoned while others are given higher priority. The overall goal of an activity, the overall purpose of doing something (such as treating patients) is, however, rarely in doubt. But the subsidiary goals, corresponding to the steps on the way, may well be, just as the choice of means to reach a goal may depend on the conditions. There are always more ways than one to do something. The adjustments thus involve the substitution of means as well as the replacement of goals. An important feature of health care resilience is the organisational recognition of and support for these adjustments.

Comparable adjustments can be found at other levels of the organisation and on longer time scales; for instance, in the way the larger organisation shifts its resources and incentives. If this is done badly, it increases the need for adjustments as the sharp end, but if it is done well, it may reduce the need for 'goal sacrificing'. This is, therefore, one way in which the system can move towards a more resilient performance. It requires, however, that the blunt end – management levels – really understand the issues and appreciate the fundamental difference between WAI and WAD. Management must acknowledge that performance at the sharp end is variable and characterised by adjustments and that this is both necessary and useful. By acknowledging this, management itself becomes able to change and to adjust its performance to the more realistic view of how work is done. This may mean that the emphasis on stereotyped responses and pre-packaged solutions (cf. the Preface) is reduced and that a more realistic attitude prevails.

Since resilience, as the health care system's ability to adjust its functioning prior to, during, or following changes and disturbances, so that it can sustain required performance under both expected and unexpected conditions, can be described in terms of how well it is able to respond, to monitor, to learn, and to anticipate, the rest of this epilogue will look at each of these four abilities and how they can be improved. Indeed, Strachan (Chapter 18) explicitly does this in the case of a patient with life-threatening heart failure. The task for us is to describe how to make the health care system as a whole more resilient, based on this synthesis of the preceding chapters. For each ability we will first summarise how they are considered from a Safety-I perspective. We will then continue by presenting the recommendations from a Safety-II perspective. This will provide some guidance on how the resilience of the care system can be improved by specific steps.

Respond

When something happens, it is important to be able to respond to expected and unexpected conditions alike so that the system is able to continue functioning. In a hospital, it is especially important to be able also quickly to adjust to situations that are new or different from what was expected.

A Safety-I perspective focuses on risks and threats, on situations where something goes wrong. If nothing goes wrong, then work can proceed according to procedures and plans, and even be optimised. The ability to respond can be improved either by eliminating risks and threats– for instance, through a classical accident analysis followed by recommendations – or by making the system more robust and less brittle. The ability to respond can also be strengthened by preparing and training specific responses to 'regular threats' (Westrum, 2006) hoping that other threats either have been eliminated or happen so rarely that they can be disregarded. Safety-I is based upon standardisation and protocols that encourage routine expertise but militates against adaptive expertise and, in turn, against resilience. Classical responding focuses on technical skills that can be taught independently, on insistence on standardisation and prescriptive protocols.

Relying on prepared responses is an advantage if the work situations are predictable, but becomes a disadvantage if the work situations are unpredictable. From a Safety-II perspective, the ability to respond must therefore take into account the unpredictability of the everyday working environment. It requires the ability to adjust the prepared responses – and to improvise. This can be nurtured by an organisational environment that cultivates diversity and provides both exposure to, and interaction with, various socio-technical constellations and work situations, even if this goes counter to the traditional approach. This does not mean that everything should be left to the discretion of clinicians – to the autonomy of people at the sharp end. But it means that health care organisations and regulators should focus on determining areas of activity that can be routinised and standardised, and understand that other areas are best left for judgements made locally in the situation. One step towards RHC is to realise the distinction, and find practical ways to express it in practice. New regulatory activities should be designed to support and complement these operational realities and local expertise, rather than attempt to supplant them, as Macrae makes clear (Chapter 9).

One possible technique is to develop 'richer communication forms' based on the experience from other domains (e.g., Sutcliffe, Lewton and Rosenthal, 2004). While such techniques are most useful in situations where communication is an explicit part, such as handovers or complicated procedures involving several actors, the basic principle may still apply to other situations, not least if it has become a natural part of how work is done. But a word of caution is needed. As Waring notes (Chapter 4), it is not easy to reconcile natural fault-lines amongst stakeholder groups; and their sectional interests, cultural characteristics and relative power resources are hard to change.

Monitor

Most daily activities involve responding in one way or another. And responding is always better if it is prepared. The ability to respond is, therefore, supported by, and may often depend on, the ability to monitor. Clearly, effective monitoring allows people to be prepared for what may happen, hence to be more effective in how they respond – either by being able to respond faster, by having the right equipment and resources (including human resources), by suspending less urgent activities, etc.

The ability to monitor means knowing how to look for that which is or can become an issue in the near term; for instance, in the sense that it may require a response of some kind. The monitoring must cover both that which happens in the environment and that which happens in the system itself, i.e. its own performance.

A Safety-I perspective does not put much emphasis on monitoring, but relies instead on standardisation and the elimination of variability. If monitoring is advocated, it usually means keeping an eye on a limited set of indicators, often supported (purportedly) by automated alarm and alert systems, or data reporting which is often delayed or out of date. Monitoring looks for things that go wrong, for deviations, for non-compliance. Monitoring is limited to what is essential for the specific process, hence excludes what may be important in a more system-wide concern. It is usually also done in the longer term, illustrated by the Global Trigger Tool and the Standardised Hospital Mortality Rate, or through accreditation.

From a Safety-II perspective, monitoring is not just looking out for things that could go wrong (warning signals), but also keeping an eye on developments that seem to go well. Monitoring thus entails learning from how things are being done well to notice the signs that can be used effectively to trim or improve performance adjustments. It requires learning from what goes right, and knowing what to look for there. In order to be effective, performance adjustments require constant monitoring. In the absence of that, everything is a surprise and the system is forced into a reactive mode, which may be unsustainable in the long term.

In order to monitor, one must know what to look for. In everyday work situations people learn rather quickly what that is by learning from their colleagues and observing the social interaction at work. But in situations that are unique, such as organisational changes, monitoring must be explicitly organised. Before introducing a change to make system performance more resilient, one should consider 'modelling changes' to identify adverse interactions and sticking points. This means that one must be prepared for what to monitor, not simply choose the things that attract attention (such as failures). One important lesson for introducing RHC is to consider metrics of safety before making a system change. In other words, you must know what and how to observe before you begin to do something.

Learn

A resilient system can adjust its way of functioning prior to, during, and *following* expected and unexpected events. The latter is, of course, the ability to learn in the sense of making use of the experiences of the past to improve how it performs in the present – and will perform in the future. It is learning form experience, in particular how to learn the right lessons from the right experience – successes as well as failures.

From a Safety-I perspective, learning is simple. Look for what went wrong, try to find the causes, and find ways to avoid a repetition. (This also means that the more serious an event is, the more there is to learn.) Since the causes are often described as failures or malfunctions of one type or another – such as non-compliance – the learning is to avoid that, i.e. to be compliant.

From a Safety-II perspective, the basis for learning should be what goes right and learning should be based on frequency rather than severity. Like other risk-critical industries, health care has a hard time valuing the exploration of successful practice but it clearly needs to move in that direction. One way of learning is carefully to examine 'workarounds' to find where there is a poor fit between prescribed practices and working conditions, following Wears and Vincent (Chapter 11). We should become better at understanding how things go right, and not just focus on how they sometimes go wrong. We should evaluate improvements to work in terms of how well they fail, in addition to how well they perform.

Learning is, however, not only important for primary and secondary care, but also for regulators who, among other things, function as a repository of operational experience and safe practices. They need to be better able to disseminate lessons learnt about health care systems, and ensure that they act as effective conduits for circulating new knowledge and innovations for dealing with risks, as noted by Macrae (Chapter 9). The operators strive to comply with the demands from the regulators, but if the regulators remain wedded to a Safety-I perspective, the operators will miss an important incentive to become resilient. Regulators should understand that it is necessary to allow a degree of local adaptation to suit the specifics of the organisations in which the regulatory activities, such as protocols, checklists, quality indicators and targets, are implemented. In the same way, organisations should strive to maintain standards that support the novice but do not constrain the expert.

There are several techniques that can support learning from practice and not just from failures. Appreciative Inquiry, for example, is an organisational development method that focuses on what goes well rather that what goes badly (Cooperrider and Srivastva, 1987). 'After Action Reviews' are structured approaches to debriefing that aim at determining what happened rather than at attributing blame. One example is known as Winston Churchill's debriefing protocol ('Why didn't I know? Why wasn't I told? Why didn't I ask?' and, 'Why didn't I tell what I knew?' [Weick and Sutcliffe, 2007]). In the spirit of Safety-II such reviews should, however, not only be applied to failures but also to things that work. Training programmes or workshops for system safety practitioners can also be developed in the spirit of Safety-II, as Robson shows (Chapter 16). One practical recommendation is to engage in generalised training – so that people, units, and organisations can identify pockets of expertise and use those to build repertoires of potential actions. This range of ideas and others, were teased out by Sutcliffe and Weick (Chapter 12).

Anticipate

Anticipation is the ability to know – or rather, to imagine – what to expect both in the short and the long term. In order to be resilient, it is important to have some ideas about technological and organisational developments, novel threats, and new opportunities. Although anticipation is an art rather than a science, the ideas should be articulated and argued in as much detail as possible. This may on the one hand increase the confidence of the predictions and on the other, make it easier to think of appropriate ways to monitor the situation and to prepare responses.

Since Safety-I basically is reactive, it pays little attention to anticipation (as illustrated by the WHO cycle shown in Chapter 1). At best, anticipation takes the form of linear extrapolations from past events and the calculation of failure probabilities. But in Safety-I, the anticipation is always limited to what goes wrong, and is conceptually very simple.

In Safety-II, the most important type of anticipation is that which takes place at the management level. Policy-makers and leaders need to pay attention to and be aware of the complex socio-cultural and socio-technical systems in which they work, but which they also attempt to change from within. They need to understand how to balance the need for prescriptive controls and widespread standards with the need for local level discretion, improvisation and judgement. And the management layers and clinician groups alike need better and more timely data on which to base decisions, as Clay-Williams and Braithwaite (Chapter 17) make clear.

Final Comments

It must be an overriding priority for resilient health care that solutions and improvements, not least the technological ones, make health care processes simpler rather than more complicated. When we develop new technology to improve clinical functions, we should always think about how it can be integrated with other systems and as far as possible, conduct usability testing to ensure that the change is appropriate and functional for the destined workplace.

When there are problems, and especially when there are new problems, it is always urgent to solve them. There is therefore a rush to find solutions and to implement them. However, in many cases, we only have a vague idea about how fast or well the solutions will work – or for how long, but that is another issue. This is particularly so for solutions that change the organisation in one way or the other. This lack of knowledge has two undesirable consequences. The first is that we really do not know *when* we should begin to look for results, and in some cases not even *where* we should look for results. The second, which actually follows from the first, is that we do not know when it is 'safe' to make another change, in the sense that the consequences of the two changes will not interfere with one another (as synergists or as antagonists). This should be a major concern, since resilient health care is unlikely to benefit from multiple changes, especially if a new change is made before the effects of earlier ones have had time to coalesce. The obvious recommendation – to be patient – will hardly be heeded because it clashes with the attraction of quick and effective actions. Yet, understanding what one does ought to be a required condition before actually doing it. In this case, it is better to stand still and reflect, than to march in the wrong direction – a point well made by Clay-Williams

(Chapter 10). Unless we have an understanding of what we are dealing with, including some reasonable assumptions about how it works (what works, when, how fast, etc.), then any kind of safety management is impossible – even Safety-I.

We would like to make perfectly clear that we do not recommend that stakeholders should do ever more thorough, more detailed, Taylorist planning. Our message is not that people should plan ever more carefully in the traditional way, which only leads to analysis paralysis. Our message is that they rather spend more time on understanding WAD. This can be done by engaging the appropriate expertise to illuminate everyday actions that get things right, to develop more skills at identifying and managing (including taking advantage of) the inevitable unexpected outcomes, and to focus less on what is easy to measure or what goes wrong. Repenning and Sterman (2001) made the same argument in the aphoristic title of their paper 'Nobody ever gets credit for fixing problems that never happened.' Yet it is also true that fixing problems that never happened is a very good thing. If Safety-II is embraced more wholeheartedly, and people in the system recognise that learning from everyday activities and things that go right is key to health care resilience, then we will be on the path to building systems where fewer problems happen. And everyone who contributes – patients, clinicians, managers, and policy-makers – can share the credit.

The bottom line is that the health care organisation, or the health care system, should understand its own goals and understand the distinction between Safety-I and Safety-II at all levels. If resilient health care can follow this advice, it may – because it is not hampered by the history and legacy of other industries – become a *de facto* leader rather than a hapless follower.

Bibliography

Adger, W.N., et al. (2002). Migration, remittances, livelihood trajectories, and social resilience. *Ambio*, 32, 921–31.

Agency for Healthcare Research and Quality. (2008). *Patient Safety Indicators Composite Measure Workgroup (final report)*. Online at http://www.qualityindicators.ahrq.gov/Downloads/Modules/PSI/PSI%20Composite%20Development.pdf, accessed 18 June 2012.

Agency for Healthcare Research and Quality. (2011). RFA-11-198. Understanding clinical information needs and health care decision making processes in the context of health information technology. Online at http://grants.nih.gov/grants/guide/pa-files/PA-11-198.html, accessed 24 November 2012.

Alderson, D.L. and Doyle, J.C. (2010). Contrasting views of complexity and their implications for network-centric infrastructures. *IEEE Transactions on Systems, Man, and Cybernetics – Part A: Systems and Humans*, 40(4), 839.

Allen, D. (2000). Doing occupational demarcation – The 'boundary-work' of nurse managers in a district general hospital. *Journal of Contemporary Ethnography*, 29(3), 326–56.

Alter, N. (2007). *Sociologie du monde du travail*. Paris: PUF, Quadrige.

Amalberti, R. (2006). Optimum system safety and optimum system resilience: Agonist or antagonists concepts? In E. Hollnagel, D. Woods and N. Leveson (eds), (2006) *Resilience Engineering: Concepts and Precepts*. Aldershot, UK: Ashgate, pp. 238–56.

Amalberti, R. (2013). *Navigating Safety, Necessary Compromises and Trade-offs – Theory and Practice*. Berlin: Springer Verlag.

Amalberti, R., et al. (2005). Five system barriers to achieving ultrasafe health care. *Annals of Internal Medicine*, 142(9), 756–64.

Amalberti, R., et al. (2006). Violations and migrations in healthcare: A framework for understanding and management. *Quality & Safety in Health Care*, 15, i66–71.

Amalberti, R., et al. (2011). Adverse events in medicine: Easy to count, complicated to understand, and complex to prevent. *Journal of Biomedical Informatics*, 44(3), 390–94.

Anders, S., et al. (2006). Limits on adaptation: Modeling resilience and brittleness in hospital emergency departments. In E. Hollnagel and E. Rigaud (eds), *Proceedings of the Second International Symposium on Resilience Engineering*. Juan-les-Pins, France, 8–10 November.Nov. 8-10.

Andrews, C. and Millar, S. (2005). Don't fumble the handoff. *MAG Mutual Healthcare Risk Manager*, 11(28), 1–2.

Antonio, G.E., Griffith, J.F. and Ahuja, A.T. (2004). Aftermath of SARS. In A.T. Ahuja and C.G.C. Ooi (eds), *Imaging in SARS*. Cambridge: Cambridge University Press (pp. 159–64).

Argyris, C. (1999). *On Organizational Learning* (2nd edition). Oxford: Wiley-Blackwell.

Argyris, C. (2010). *Organizational Traps: Leadership, Culture, Organizational Design*. New York: Oxford University Press.

Arnold, J.M., et al. (2006). Canadian Cardiovascular Society consensus conference recommendations on heart failure 2006: Diagnosis and management. *Canadian Journal of Cardiology*, 22, 23–45.

Ashby, W.R. (1956). *An Introduction to Cybernetics*. London: Chapman-Hall.

Ashby, W.R. (1958). Requisite variety and its implications for the control of complex systems. *Cybernetica*, 1, 83–99.

Austin, W. (2007). The ethics of everyday practice: Healthcare environments as moral communities. *Advances in Nursing Science*, 30(1), 81–8.

Axelrod, R. and Cohen, M.D. (2000). *Harnessing Complexity: Organizational Implications of a Scientific Frontier*. New York, NY: Basic Books (pp. 43, 157).

Bagian, J. (2007). Discussion about the challenge of training healthcare workers to solve novel problems and understand systems thinking. (Personal communication, March 2007.)

Baker, G.R. and Norton, P. (2001). Making patients safer! Reducing error in Canadian healthcare. *Healthcare Papers*, 2(1), 10–31.

Baker, G. R., et al. (2004). The Canadian adverse events study: The incidence of adverse events among hospital patients in Canada. *Canadian Medical Association Journal*, 170(11), 1,678–86.

Barnato, A.E., et al. (2007). Communication and decision making in cancer care: Setting research priorities for decision support / patients' decision aids. *Medical Decision Making*, 27, 625–34.

Barnes, B. (2001). The macro / micro problem of structure and agency. In G. Ritzer and B. Smart (eds), *Handbook of Social Theory*. Thousand Oaks, CA: Sage (pp. 339–52).

Baron, R.M. and Misovich, S.J. (1999). On the relationship between social and cognitive modes of organization. In S. Chaiken and Y. Trope (eds), *Dual-process Theories in Social Psychology*. S. Chaiken and Y. Trope. New York: The Guilford Press (pp. 586–605).

Baroody, A.J. and Rosu, L. (2006). Adaptive expertise with basic addition and subtraction combinations – The number sense view. Paper presented at the Annual Meeting of the American Educational Research Association. San Francisco, CA, April.

Bates, D.W. and Gawande, A.A. (2003). Improving safety with information technology. *New England Journal of Medicine*, 348(25), 2,526–34.

Beattie, J. and Goodlin, S. (eds), (2008). *Supportive Care in Heart Failure*. Oxford: Oxford University Press.

Belkin, L. (1997). Getting past blame: How can we save the next victim? *New York Times Sunday Magazine*. 15 June.

Bender, K., et al. (2007). Capacity for survival: Exploring strengths of homeless street youth. *Child Youth Care Forum*, 36(1), 25–42.

Bertalanffy, L. von (1973). *General System Theory: Foundations, Development, Applications*. Harmondsworth: Penguin.

Berwick, D.M. (2003). Improvement, trust, and the healthcare workforce. *Quality and Safety in Health Care*, 12(6), 448–52.

Bhamra, R., Dani, S. and Burnard, K. (2011). Resilience: The concept, a literature review and future directions. *International Journal of Production Research*, 49(18), 5,375–93.

Bigley, G.A. and Roberts, K.H. (2001). The incident command system: Organizing for high reliability in complex and unpredictable environments. *Academy of Management Journal*, 44(6), 1,281–99.

Blatt, R., et al. (2006). A sensemaking lens on reliability. *Journal of Organizational Behavior*, 27, 897–917.

Blavier A., et al. (2007). Comparison of learning curves in classical and robotic laparoscopy according to the viewing condition. *American Journal of Surgery*, 194, 115–21.

Bolman, L.G. and Deal, T.E. (2008). *Reframing Organizations: Artistry, Choice, and Leadership* (4th Edition). San Francisco: Jossey-Bass Publishing.

Boyd, K. and Murray, S.A. (2010). Recognising and managing key transitions in end of life care. *British Medical Journal*, 341, 649–52.

Bradley, E.H., et al. (2011). Health and social services expenditures: Associations with health outcomes. *British Medical Journal Quality and Safety*, 20(10), 826–31.

Braithwaite, J. (2005). Hunter-gatherer human nature and health system safety: An evolutionary cleft stick? *International Journal for Quality in Health Care*, 17(6), 541–5.

Braithwaite, J. (2006). Analysing structural and cultural change in acute settings using a Giddens-Weick paradigmatic approach. *Health Care Analysis*, 14(2), 91–102. [7, 11]

Braithwaite, J. (2010). Between-group behaviour in health care: Gaps, edges, boundaries, disconnections, weak ties, spaces and holes. A systematic review. *BMC Health Services Research*. Online at http://www.biomedcentral.com/1472-6963/10/330, accessed 29 August 2012.

Braithwaite, J. and Clay-Williams, R. (2012). Mandating health care by creeps and jerks. *International Journal for Quality in Health Care*, 24(3), 197–9.

Braithwaite, J. and Coiera, E. (2010). Beyond patient safety Flatland. *Journal of the Royal Society of Medicine*, 103(6), 219–25.

Braithwaite, J. and Westbrook, M. (2005). Rethinking clinical organisational structures: An attitude survey of doctors, nurses and allied health staff in clinical directorates. *Journal of Health Services and Research Policy*, 10(1), 10–17.

Braithwaite, J., Hyde, P. and Pope, C. (2010). *Culture and Climate in Health Care Organizations*. Basingstoke: Palgrave Macmillan.

Braithwaite, J., Runciman, W.B. and Merry, A.F. (2009). Towards safer, better healthcare: Harnessing the natural properties of complex sociotechnical systems. *Quality and Safety in Health Care*, 18(1), 37–41.

Braithwaite, J., Vining, R. and Lazarus, L. (1994). The boundaryless hospital. *Australian and New Zealand Journal of Medicine*, 24(5), 565–71.

Braithwaite, J., Westbrook, J. and Iedema, R. (2005). Restructuring as gratification. *Journal of the Royal Society of Medicine*, 98(12), 542–4.

Braithwaite, J., et al. (2006). Experiences of health professionals who conducted root cause analyses after undergoing a safety improvement programme. *Quality and Safety in Health Care*, 15(6), 393.

Braithwaite, J., et al. (2007). Are health systems changing in support of patient safety? A multi-methods evaluation of education, attitudes and practice. *International Journal of Health Care Quality Assurance*, 20(7), 585–601.

Braithwaite, J., et al. (2010). Cultural and other associated enablers, and barriers, to adverse incident reporting. *Quality and Safety in Health Care*, 19, 229–33.

Braithwaite, J., et al. (2013). Continuing differences between health professions' attitudes: The saga of accomplishing systems-wide interprofessionalism. *International Journal of Quality in Healthcare*. 25(1), 8-15.

Bratzler, D., et al. (2005). Use of antimicrobial prophylaxis for major surgery. *Arch Surg*, *140*, 174-82.

Brennan, T.A. and Berwick D.M. (1996). *New Rules: Regulation, Markets and the Quality of American Health Care*. San Francisco: Jossey-Bass.

Brennan, T.A., et al. (1991). Incidence of adverse events and negligence in hospitalized patients: Results of the Harvard Medical Practice Study I. *New England Journal of Medicine*, 324, 370–76.

Bressolle, M.C., et al. (1996). Traitement cognitif et organisationnel des micro-incidents dans le domaine du contrôle aérien: Analyse des boucles de régulation formelles et informelles. In G. de Terssac and E. Friedberg (eds), *Coopération et conception* G. De Terssac and E. Friedberg. Toulouse: Octares (pp. 267–88).

Buntin, M.B., et al. (2011). The benefits of health information technology: A review of the recent literature shows predominantly positive results. *Health Affairs*, 30(3), 464–71.

Burnett, S., et al. (2010). Organisational readiness: Exploring the preconditions for success in organisation-wide patient safety improvement programmes. *Quality and Safety in Health Care*, 19(4), 313–17.

Camillus, J.C. (1982). Reconciling logical incrementalism and synoptic formalism – an integrated approach to designing strategic planning processes. *Strategic Management Journal*, 3(3), 277–83.

Campbell, D.T. (1990). Asch's moral epistemology for socially shared knowledge. In I. Rock (ed.), *The Legacy of Solomon Asch: Essays In Cognition and Social Psychology*. Hillsdale, NJ: Erlbaum (pp. 39–52).

Card, A.J., Ward, J.R. and Clarkson, P.J. (2011). *Risk Control after Root Cause Analysis: A Systematic Literature Review*. Online at http://cambridge.academia.edu/AlanCard/Papers/440766/Risk_Control_after_Root_Cause_Analysis_A_Systematic_Literature_Review, accessed 12 June 2012.

Card, A.J., Ward, J.R. and Clarkson, P.J. (2012). Successful risk analysis may not always lead to successful risk control: A systematic review of the risk control literature. *Journal of Healthcare Risk Management*, 31(3), 6–12.

Cardiff, K. (2007). *Is Quality Safety? Is Safety Quality?* M.Sc. Lund University. [online] Lund University Master's Program in Human Factors and System Safety. Online at http://www.leonardo.lth.se/education/masters_program/masters_theses/, accessed 30 July 2012.

Carthey, J., Chandra, V. and Loosemore, M. (2008). Assessing the adaptive capacity of hospital facilities to cope with climate-related extreme weather events: A risk management approach. *Association of Researchers in Construction Management*, 742–57.

Carthey, J., Chandra, V. and Loosemore, M. (2009). Adapting Australian health facilities to cope with climate-related extreme weather events. *Journal of Facilities Management*, 7(1), 36–51.

Carthey, J., de Leval, M.R. and Reason, J.T. (2001). Institutional resilience in healthcare systems. *Quality in Health Care*, 10, 29–32.

Carthey, J., et al. (2011). Breaking the rules: Understanding non-compliance with policies and guidelines, *British Medical Journal*, 343–7.

Cassel, C.K. and Guest, J.A. (2012). Choosing wisely: Helping physicians and patients make smart decisions about their care. *Jama*, 307(17), 1, 801–2.

Cerulo, K.A. (2006). *Never Saw It Coming: Cultural Challenges to Envisioning the Worst*. Chicago: University of Chicago Press.

Chang, A., et al. (2005). The JCAHO patient safety event taxonomy: A standardized terminology and classification schema for near misses and adverse events. *International Journal for Quality in Health Care*, 17(2), 92–105.

Chaudhry, S.I., et al. (2007). Patterns of weight change preceding hospitalization for heart failure. *Circulation*, 116, 1,549–54.

Chemin, C., et al. (2010). *Projet CLHOE: Interactions Individus-Collectif-Organisation dans un Service de Soins Intensifs*. Actes du 45° Congrès de la Société d'Ergonomie de Langue Française (SELF) 'Fiabilité, Résilience et Adaptation', Liège.

Christianson, M.K. and Sutcliffe, K.M. (2009). Sensemaking, high reliability organizing, and resilience. In P. Croskerry, et al. (eds), *Patient Safety in Emergency Medicine*. P. Croskerry, K. Cosby, S. Schenkel and R. Wears. Philadelphia, PA: Lippincott Williams and Wilkins (pp. 27–33).

Chuang, S.W. (2012). *Standardization versus Adaptation for Patient Safety: A Lesson Learnt from Three Scabies Outbreaks. Resilient Health Care Net Symposium*, Middelfart, Denmark, 3 June 2012.

Chuang, S.W. and Howley P. (2012). Beyond root cause analysis: An enriched system oriented event analysis model for wide applications. *System Engineering*, 16(3), DOI 10.1002/sys.21246.

Chuang, S.W., Howley, P. and Lin, S.H. (2011). *Beyond the Root Cause Analysis: The Cessation of Scabies Outbreaks by the Application of an Enriched System-Oriented Events Analysis Mode*. ISQua 28th International Conference, Hong Kong, 14–17 September.

Chun, S., et al. (2012). Lifetime analysis of hospitalizations and survival of patients newly admitted with heart failure. *Circulation Heart Failure*, 5(4), 414–21.

Cilliers, P. (1998). *Complexity and Postmodernism*. London and New York: Routledge.

Cimellaro, G.P., Reinhorn, A.M. and Bruneau, M. (2010). Seismic resilience of a hospital system. *Structure and Infrastructure Engineering*, 6(1–2), 127–44.

Clot, Y. (2010). *Le travail à cœur. Pour en finir avec les risques psychosociaux*. Paris: La Découverte.

Cohen, A., et al. (2008). Venous thromboembolism risk and prophylaxis in the acute hospital care setting (ENDORSE study): A multinational cross-sectional. *Lancet*. 371(9,610), 387–94.

Collingridge, D. (1996). Resilience, flexibility, and diversity in managing the risks of technologies. In C. Hood and D.K.C. Jones (eds), *Accident and Design: Contemporary Debates on Risk Management*. London: Taylor and Francis.

Comfort, L.K., Boin, A. and Demchak, C.C. (eds), (2010). *Designing Resilience: Preparing for Extreme Events*. Pittsburgh: University of Pittsburgh.

Cook, R.I. (1998). *Being Bumpable: The Complexity of ICU Operations and their Consequences* (CTL Report 98–01). Chicago, IL: Cognitive Technologies Laboratory, University of Chicago.

Cook, R.I. (2012). Discussion about the application of Lean methodology in healthcare (Personal communication, May 2012).

Cook, R.I. and Nemeth, C.P. (2010). 'Those found responsible have been sacked': Some observations on the usefulness of error. *Cognition Technology & Work*, 12, 87–93.

Cook, R.I. and Rasmussen, J. (2005). 'Going solid': A model of system dynamics and consequences for patient safety. *Quality and Safety in Health Care*, 14(2), 130.

Cook, R.I. and Woods, D.D. (1994). Operating at the sharp end: The complexity of human error. In M.S. Bogner (ed.), *Human Error in Medicine*. Hillsdale, NJ: Lawrence Erlbaum Associates, 255–310.

Cook, R.I., Render, M. and Woods, D.D. (2000). Gaps in the continuity of care and progress on patient safety. *British Medical Journal*, 320(7,237), 791–94.

Cook, R.I., Woods, D.D. and Miller, C. (1998). *A Tale of Two Stories: Contrasting Views of Patient Safety*. Report from a Workshop on Assembling the Scientific Basis for Progress on Patient Safety. Chicago: National Patient Safety Foundation.

Cooperrider, D.L. and Srivastva, S. (1987). Appreciative inquiry in organizational life. *Research in Organizational Change and Development*, 1(1), 129–69.

Costantino, C.A. and Merchant, C.S. (1996). *Designing Conflict Management Systems*. San Francisco: Jossey-Bass Publishers.

Degos, L., et al. (2009). The frontiers of patient safety: Breaking the traditional mold. *British Medical Journal*, (338), b2,585.

Dekker, S.W.A. (2006a). *The Field Guide to Understanding Human Error*. Aldershot, UK: Ashgate.

Dekker, S.W.A. (2006b). Resilience engineering: Chronicling the emergence of confused consensus. In E. Hollnagel, D.D. Woods and N. Leveson (eds), *Resilience Engineering: Concepts and Precepts* E. Hollnagel, D. D. Woods and N. Leveson. Aldershot, UK: Ashgate (p. 82).

Dekker, S.W.A. (2007). Discussion about the failure of reductionistic models to fully explain failure and safety in complex systems such as health care (Personal communication, October 2007).

Dekker, S.W.A. (2011a). *Drift into Failure: From Hunting Broken Components to Understanding Complex Systems*. Farnham, UK: Ashgate.

Dekker, S.W.A. (2011b). *Patient Safety: A Human Factors Approach*. Boca Raton, FL: CRC Press.

Dekker, S.W.A., Cilliers, P. and Hofmeyr, J.-H. (2011). The complexity of failure: Implications of complexity theory for safety investigations, *Safety Science*, 49, 939–45.

Dekker, S.W.A., et al. (2008). *Resilience Engineering: New Directions for Measuring and Maintaining Safety in Complex Systems* (final report). Sweden: Lund University School of Aviation.

Dekker, S.W.A., Nyce, J. and Myers, D. (2012). The little engine who could not: 'Rehabilitating' the individual in safety research. *Cognition, Technology & Work* (in press).

Department of Health (2000). *An Organisation with a Memory*. London: TSO.

Dimov, D.P., Shepherd, D.A. and Sutcliffe, K.M. (2007). Requisite expertise, firm reputation and status in venture capital investment allocation decisions. *Journal of Business Venturing*, 22, 481–502.

Dixon Woods, M., et al. (2011). Problems and promises of innovation: Why healthcare needs to rethink its love / hate relationship with the new. *British Medical Journal Quality and Safety*, 20, i47–i51.

Donaldson, L. (2009). An international language for patient safety: Global progress in patient safety requires classification of key concepts. *International Journal for Quality in Health Care*, 2, 1.

Douglas, M. (1994). *Risk and Blame: Essays in Cultural Theory*. London: Routledge.

Dwyer, J. (2012). An infection, unnoticed, turns unstoppable. *The New York Times*. 11 July, A15.

Eddy, D.M. (1990). Clinical decision making: From theory to practice. Designing a practice policy. Standards, guidelines, and options. *Journal of the American Medical Association*, 263(22), 3,077, 3,081, 3,084.

Edmondson, A.C. (2003). Speaking up in the operating room: How team leaders promote learning in interdisciplinary action teams. *Journal of Management Studies*, 40(6), 1,419–52.

Eljiz, K., Fitzgerald, A. and Sloan, T. (2010). Interpersonal relationships and decision-making about patient flow: What and who really matters? In J. Braithwaite, P. Hyde and C. Pope (eds), *Culture and Climate in Health Care Organizations* J. Braithwaite, P. Hyde and C. Pope. Basingstoke: Palgrave Macmillan, 70–81.

Ellis, B. and Herbert, S.I. (2011). Complex adaptive systems (CAS): An overview of key elements, characteristics and application to management theory. *Informatics in Primary Care*, 19(1), 33–7.

Evidence-Based Medicine Working Group. (1992). Evidence-based medicine. A new approach to teaching the practice of medicine. *Journal of the American Medical Association*, 268.

Faverge, J.-M. (1979–1980). Le travail en tant qu'activité de récupération. *Bulletin de Psychologie*, XXXIII(344), 203–6.

Feltovich, P.J., Spiro, R.J. and Coulson, R.L. (1997). Issues of expert flexibility in contexts characterized by complexity and change. In P.J. Feltovich, K.M. Ford and R.R. Hoffman (eds), *Expertise in Context: Human and Machine*. Menlo Park, CA: AAAI Press.

Fitzsimons, D. and Strachan, P.H. (2012). Overcoming the challenges of conducting research with people who have advanced heart failure and palliative care needs. *European Journal of Cardiovascular Nursing*, 11(2), 248–54.

Flin, R. (2007). Measuring safety culture in healthcare: A case for accurate diagnosis. *Safety Science*, 45(6), 653–67.

Foley, M. (2011). *Future Arrangements for Governance of NSW Health: Report of the Director-General*. Sydney: NSW Government.

Fox, R. (1980). The evolution of uncertainty. *Milbank Quarterly*, 58(1), 1–49.

Frank, A.W. (2010). *Letting Stories Breath – A Socio-Narratology*. Chicago and London: University of Chicago Press.

Frankovich, J., Longhurst, C.A. and Sutherland, S.M. (2011). Evidence-based medicine in the EMR era. *New England Journal of Medicine*, 365(19), 1,758–9.

Fraser, S.W. and Greenhalgh, T. (2001). Coping with complexity: Educating for capability. *British Medical Journal*, 323, 799–803.

Fredrickson, B.L. (2002). Positive emotions. In C.R. Snyder and S.J. Lopez (eds), *Handbook of Positive Psychology*. New York: Oxford University Press (pp. 120–34).

Fredrickson, B.L., et al. (2003). *Journal of Personality and Social Psychology*, 84(2), 365–76.

Freidson, E. (1970). *The Profession of Medicine*. London: University of Chicago Press.

Gabbay, J. and May, A. (2004). Evidence based guidelines or collectively constructed 'mindlines?' Ethnographic study of knowledge management in primary care. *British Medical Journal*, 329(7,473), 1,013.

Gabriel, Y. (2008). *Organizing Words: A Thesaurus for Social and Organizational Studies*. Oxford: Oxford University Press.

Gagnon, M.P., et al. (2012). Systematic review of factors influencing the adoption of information and communication technologies by healthcare professionals. *Journal of Medical Systems*, 36(1), 241.

Garling, P. (2008). *Final Report of the Special Commission of Inquiry: Acute Care Services in NSW Public Hospitals*. Sydney: NSW Government.

Gawande, A. (2012). Failure and rescue. *The New Yorker* [online 4 June]. Online at http://www.newyorker.com/online/blogs/newsdesk/2012/06/atul-gawande-failure-and-rescue.html, accessed 25 September 2012.

Geary, D.C. (2003). Arithmetical development: Commentary on Chapters 9 through 15 and future directions. In A.J. Baroody and A. Dowker (eds), *The Development of Arithmetic Concepts and Skills: Constructing Adaptive Expertise*. Mahwah, NJ: Lawrence Erlbaum Associates (pp. 453–64).

Gergen, K. (2009). *An Invitation to Social Constructionism*. London: Sage.

Ghaferi, A.A., Birkmeyer, J.D. and Dimick, J.B. (2009a). Variation in hospital mortality associated with inpatient surgery. *The New England Journal of Medicine*, 361(14), 1,368–74.

Ghaferi, A.A., Birkmeyer, J.D. and Dimick, J.B. (2009b). Complications, failure to rescue, and mortality with major inpatient surgery in medicare patients. *Annals of Surgery*, 250(6), 1,029–34.

Giannone, D., Reichlin, L. and Small, D. (2008). Nowcasting: The real-time informational content of macroeconomic data. *Journal of Monetary Economics*, 55(4), 665–76.

Gibb, R.W. and Olson, W. (2008). Classification of Air Force aviation accidents: Mishap trends and prevention. *The International Journal of Aviation Psychology*, 18(4), 305–25.

Gleick, J. (1987). *Chaos: Making a New Science*. New York. Penguin Books.

Goldfinch, S. (2007). Pessimism, computer failure, and information systems development in the public sector. *Public Administration Review*, 67(5), 917–29.

Golding, N. (2012). Accountability probe could lead to regulation for managers. *Health Service Journal*. Online at http://www.hsj.co.uk/news/policy/accountability-probe-could-lead-to-regulation-for-managers/5050422.article, [accessed 29 October 2012].

Goldmann, D. (2006). System failure versus personal accountability – the case for clean hands. *New England Journal of Medicine*, 355, 121–3.

Goodlin, S.J., et al. (2004). Consensus statement: Palliative and supportive care in advanced heart failure. *Journal of Cardiac Failure, 10*(3), 200-209.

Grabowski, M.R., et al. (2007). Accident precursors and safety nets: Initial results from the Leading Indicators of Safety Project. ABS Technical Papers 2007. Presented at SNAME, Ft. Lauderdale, Florida, November 2007. Available at http://www.eagle.org/eagleExternalPortalWEB/ShowProperty/BEA%20Repository/References/Technical%20Papers/2007/AccidentPrecursors, accessed 18 October 2012.

Greenberg, M.D., et al. (2010). *Is Better Patient Safety Associated with Less Malpractice Activity?* Available at http://www.rand.org/pubs/technical_reports/2010/RAND_TR824.pdf, accessed 22 June 2012.

Greenhalgh, J., et al. (2012). How do doctors refer to patient-reported outcome measures (PROMS) in oncology consultations? *Quality of Life Research* [Epub ahead of print].

Grote, G. (2006). Rules management as source for loose coupling in high-risk systems. *Proceedings of the 2nd Symposium on Resilience Engineering*, Juan-les-Pins, France. Online at http://www.resilience-engineering.org/, accessed 31 August 2012.

Grothberg, E. (1995). *A Guide to Promoting Resilience in Children: Strengthening the Human Spirit*. Den Haag: Bernard van Leer Foundation.

Guldenmund, F. (2000). The nature of safety culture: A review of theory and research. *Safety Science*, 34(1), 215–57.

Gunderson, L.H. and Holling, C.S. (2002). *Panarchy: Understanding Transformations in Human and Natural Systems*. Washington, DC: Island Press.

Hacking, I. (1999). *The Social Construction of What?* Cambridge: Harvard University Press.

Hass, M. and Graydon, K. (2009). Sources of resiliency among successful foster youth. *Children and Youth Services Review*, 31, 457–63.

Hatano, G. (1982). Cognitive consequences of practice in culture specific procedural skills. *The Quarterly Newsletter of the Laboratory of Comparative Human Cognition*, 4, 15–18.

Hatano, G. and Inagaki K. (1984). The two courses of expertise. *Research and Clinical Center for Child Development Annual Report*, 6, 27–36.

Hatano, G. and Oura, Y. (2003). Reconceptualizing school learning using insight from expertise research. *Educational Researcher*, 32(8), 26–9.

Hayes, R.H. and Wheelwrite, S.C. (1979a). Linking manufacturing process and product life cycle. *Harvard Business Review*, 57, 133–40.

Hayes, R.H. and Wheelwrite, S.C. (1979b). The dynamics of process-product lifecycles. *Harvard Business Review*, 57, 127–36.

Haynes, A.B., et al. (2011). Changes in safety attitude and relationship to decreased postoperative morbidity and mortality following implementation of a checklist-based surgical safety intervention. *BMJ Quality and Safety*, 20(1), 102–7.

Heckman, G.A., et al. (2007). Heart failure in older persons. *Canadian Journal of General Internal Medicine*, 2, 24–6.

Heinrich, H.W. (1931). *Industrial Accident Prevention: A Scientific Approach*. New York: McGraw-Hill.

Henriksen, K. and Kaplan H. (2003). Hindsight bias, outcome knowledge and adaptive learning. *Quality and Safety in Health Care*, 12(2, Suppl.), 46–50.

Heyland, D.K., et al. (2006). What matters most in end-of-life care: Perceptions of seriously ill patients and their family members; Canadian Researchers End-of-Life Network (CARENET). *Canadian Medical Association Journal*, 174(5), 627–33.

Hillman, K., et al. (2005). Introduction of the medical emergency team (MET) system: A cluster-randomised controlled trial. *Lancet*, 365(9,477), 2,091–7.

Hindle, D., et al. (2006). Patient safety: A comparative analysis of eight inquiries in five countries. *Centre for Clinical Governance Research Monograph*. Sydney, Australia: University of New South Wales.

Hoffman, J. (2007). CRICO's handoff-related malpractice cases. *Forum*, 25, 1–21.

Hoffman, R.R. and Woods, D.D. (2011). Beyond Simon's slice: Five fundamental trade-offs that bound the performance of macrocognitive work systems. *IEEE Intelligent Systems*, 26(6), 67–71.

Holling, C.S. (1996). Engineering resilience versus ecological resilience. In P. Schulze (ed.), *Engineering Within Ecological Constraints*. Washington, DC: National Academy Press (pp. 31–44).

Hollnagel, E. (1993). *Human Reliability Analysis: Context and Control*. London: Academic Press.

Hollnagel, E. (2004). *Barriers and Accident Prevention*. Aldershot, UK: Ashgate.

Hollnagel, E. (2008). Investigation as an impediment to learning. In E. Hollnagel, C.P. Nemeth and S.W.A. Dekker (eds), *Remaining Sensitive to the Possibility of Failure*. Aldershot, UK: Ashgate (pp. 259–68).

Hollnagel, E. (2009a). *The ETTO Principle: Efficiency-Thoroughness Trade-Off. Why Things that Go Right Sometimes Go Wrong*. Aldershot, UK: Ashgate.

Hollnagel, E. (2009b). The four cornerstones of resilience engineering. In C.P. Nemeth, E. Hollnagel and S.W.A. Dekker (eds), *Resilience Engineering Perspectives: Preparation and Restoration*. Aldershot, UK: Ashgate (pp. 117–33, 177).

Hollnagel, E. (2011a). *The ETTO Principle. Efficiency-Thoroughness Trade-Off or Why Things that Go Right Sometimes Go Wrong*. Farnham, UK: Ashgate.

Hollnagel, E. (2011b). Prologue: The scope of resilience engineering. In E. Hollnagel, J. Pariès, D.D. Woods and J. Wreathall (eds), *Resilience Engineering in Practice: A Guidebook*. Farnham, UK: Ashgate (pp. xxix–xxxix).

Hollnagel, E. (2012). *FRAM: The Functional Resonance Analysis Method*. Farnham, UK: Ashgate.

Hollnagel, E. (ed.) (2010). *Safer Complex Industrial Environments*. Boca Raton, FL: CRC Press.

Hollnagel, E. and Woods, D.D. (2005). *Joint Cognitive Systems: Foundations of Cognitive Systems Engineering*. Boca Raton, FL: CRC Press.

Hollnagel, E., Nemeth, C.P. and Dekker, S.W.A. (eds), (2008). *Resilience Engineering: Remaining Sensitive to the Possibility of Failure*. Aldershot, UK: Ashgate.

Hollnagel, E. et al. (eds), (2010). *Resilience Engineering in Practice: A Guidebook*. Farnham, UK: Ashgate.

Hollnagel, E., Woods, D.D. and Leveson, N. (eds), (2006). *Resilience Engineering: Concepts and Precepts*. Aldershot, UK: Ashgate.

Hood, C., Rothstein, H. and Baldwin, R. (2001). *The Government of Risk*. Oxford: Oxford University Press.

Howlett, J., et al. (2010). End of life planning in heart failure: It should be the end of the beginning. *Canadian Journal of Cardiology*, 26(3), 135–41.

Hughes, C., Travaglia, J. and Braithwaite, J. (2010). Bad stars or guiding lights? Learning from disasters to improve patient safety. *Quality and Safety in Health Care*, 19(4), 332–6.

Hutt, E., et al. (2011). Regional variation in mortality and subsequent hospitalization of nursing residents with heart failure. *Journal of the American Medical Directors Association*, 12, 585–601.

Hutter, B.M. (2001). *Regulation and Risk: Occupational Health and Safety on the Railways*. Oxford: Oxford University Press.

Iedema, R.A.M., et al. (2006). A root cause analysis: Confronting the disjunction between formal rules and situated clinical activity. *Social Science & Medicine*, 63(5), 1,201–12.

Illich, I. (1976). *Medical Nemesis: The Expropriation of Health*. New York: Random House.

Institute for Healthcare Improvement (2012). Institute for Healthcare Improvement: IHI offerings. Online at http://www.ihi.org/offerings/Pages/default.aspx, accessed 31 August 2012.

Institute of Medicine. (2012). *Health IT and Patient Safety: Building Safer Systems for Better Care*. Washington, DC: The National Academies Press.

Isaacs, W. (1999). *Dialogue and the Art of Thinking Together*. New York: Doubleday Random House.

Institute for Safe Medical Practices. (2010). Drug shortages: National survey reveals high level of frustration, low level of safety. *ISMP Medication Safety Alert*, 15, 1–3.

Jaarsma, T., et al. (2009). Palliative care in heart failure: A position statement from the palliative care workshop of the Heart Failure Association of the European Society of Cardiology. (Advanced Heart Failure Study Group of the HFA of the ESC.) *European Journal of Heart Failure*, 11, 433–43.

James, W. (1890). *The Principles of Psychology*. London: Macmillan and Co.

James, W. (1996). *Some Problems of Philosophy: A Beginning of an Introduction to Philosophy*. Lincoln, NE: University of Nebraska Press (pp. 50–51).

Jensen, V. and Rappaport, B.A. (2010). The reality of drug shortages – the case of the injectable agent propofol. *New England Journal of Medicine*, 363(9), 806–7.

Kaasalainen, S., et al. (2011). Managing palliative care for patients with advanced heart failure. *Canadian Journal of Nursing Research*, 43(3), 38–57.

Kaushal, R., Shojania, K.G. and Bates, D.W. (2003). Effects of computerized physician order entry and clinical decision support systems on medication safety: A systematic review. *Archives of Internal Medicine*, 163(12), 1,409.

Kenney, C. (2010). *Transforming Health Care: Virginia Mason Medical Center's Pursuit of the Perfect Patient Experience*. New York, NY: Productivity Press, Taylor & Francis Group.

Kernick, W. (ed.) (2004). *Complexity and Healthcare Organization*. Oxford: Radcliffe Medical Press.

Klein, G. (1998). *Sources of Power*. Boston: MIT Press.

Knorr-Cetina, K. (1981). *The Manufacture of Knowledge: An Essay on the Constructivist and Contextual Nature of Science*. London: Pergamon Press.

Knox, G.E., Simpson, K.R. and Garite, T. J. (1999). High reliability perinatal units: An approach to the prevention of patient injury and medical malpractice claims. *Journal of Healthcare Risk Management*, 19(2), 24–32.

Ko, D. T., et al. (2008). Life expectancy after an index hospitalization for patients with heart failure: A population-based study. *American Heart Journal*, 155, 324–31.

Kohn, L.T., Corrigan, J.M. and Donaldson, M.S. (eds), (2000). *To Err Is Human: Building a Safer Health System*. Washington, DC: National Academy Press.

Kuhn, A.M. and Youngberg, B.J. (2002). The need for risk management to evolve to assure a culture of safety. *Quality & Safety in Health Care*, 11, 158–62.

Kumpfer, K.L. (1999). Factors and processes contributing to resilience: The positive resilience framework. In M.D. Glantz and J.L. Johnson (eds),

Resilience and Development: Positive Life Adaptions. New York: Academic / Plenum Publishers (pp. 179–224).

Lagadec, P. (1993). *Preventing Chaos in a Crisis*. New York: McGraw-Hill.

Lallement, M., et al. (2011). Maux du travail, dégradation, recomposition ou illusion? *Sociologie du travail*, 53, 3–36.

Landau, M. and Chisholm, D. (1995). The arrogance of optimism: Notes on failure avoidance management. *Journal of Contingencies and Crisis Management*, 3, 67–80.

Landrigan, C.P., et al. (2010). Temporal trends in rates of patient harm resulting from medical care. *New England Journal of Medicine*, 363, 2, 124–34.

Lang, A., et al. (2009). Broadening the safety agenda to include home care services. *Healthcare Quarterly*, 9, 124–6.

Langley, A. and Tsoukas, H. Introducing 'perspective on process organization studies'. In T. Hernes and S. Maitlis (eds), *Process, Sensemaking, and Organizing*. New York: Oxford University Press (pp. 1–26).

Latour, B. (2005). *Reassembling the Social: An Introduction to Actor-Network-Theory*. Oxford; New York: Oxford University Press.

Lave, J. and Wenger, E. (1991). *Legitimate Peripheral Participation*. Cambridge: Cambridge University Press.

Leape, L.L., et al. (1991). The nature of adverse events in hospitalized patients. Results of the Harvard Medical Practice Study II. *New England Journal of Medicine*, 324, 377–84.

LeMond, L. and Allen, L.A. (2011). Palliative care and hospice in advanced heart failure. *Progress in Cardiovascular Disease*, 54, 168–78.

Letiche, H. (2008). *Making Healthcare Care: Managing via Simple Guiding Principles*. Charlotte, NC: Information Age Publishing.

Leveson, N., et al. (2009). Moving beyond normal accidents and high reliability organizations: A systems approach to safety in complex systems. *Organization Studies*, 30(2–3), 227–49.

Lider, J. (1983). *Military Theory: Concept, Structure, Problems*. New York: St. Martin's Press.

Lindblom, C.A. (1959). The science of 'muddling through'. *Public Administration Review*, 19(2), 79–88.

Lorenz, E.N. (1993). *The Essence of Chaos*. Seattle: University of Washington Press.

Lorenz, E. (2001). Models of cognition, the contextualisation of knowledge and organisational theory. *Journal of Management and Governance*, 5(3–4), 307–30.

Low, J., et al. (2011). Palliative care in advanced heart failure: An international review of the perspectives of recipients and health professionals on care provision. *Journal of Cardiac Failure*, 17(3), 231–52.

Lundberg, J., Rollenhagen, C. and Hollnagel, E. (2009). What-You-Look-For-Is-What-You-Find – The consequence of underlying accident models in eight accident investigation manuals. *Safety Science*, 47(10), 1,297–311.

Macrae, C. (2010). Regulating resilience? Regulatory work in high-risk arenas. In B. Hutter (ed.), *Anticipating Risks and Organising Risk Regulation*. Cambridge: Cambridge University Press.

Mainz, J. (2003). Defining and classifying clinical indicators for quality improvement. *International Journal for Quality in Health Care*, 15(6), 523–30.

Maluccio, A.N. (2002). Resilience: A many-splendored construct? *American Journal of Orthopsychiatry*, 72, 596–9.

Mant, J. (2001). Process versus outcome indicators in the assessment of quality of health care. *International Journal for Quality in Health Care*, 13(6), 475–80.

Mant, J. and Hicks, N. (1995). Detecting differences in quality of care: The sensitivity of measures of process and outcome in treating acute myocardial infarction. *British Medical Journal*, 311, 793–9.

Marcella, J., et al. (2012). Understanding organizational context and heart failure management in long term care homes in Ontario, Canada. *Health*, 4(9), 725–34.

Martin, J. (2002). *Organizational Culture: Mapping the Terrain*. Thousand Oaks, CA: Sage.

Maslow, A.H. (1943). A theory of human motivation. *Psychological Review*, 50(4), 370–96.

Masten, A. and Wright, M.O. (2010). Resilience over the lifespan: Developmental perspectives on resistance, recovery, and transformation. In J. Reich, A.J. Zautra and J. Hall (eds), *Handbook of Adult Resilience*. New York: The Guilford Press (pp. 213–23).

Mathe, J.L., et al. (2009). A model-integrated, guideline-driven, clinical decision-support system. *IEEE Software*, 26(4), 54–61.

McDonald, R., Waring, J. and Harrison, S. (2006). Rules, safety and the narrativisation of identity: A hospital operating theatre case study. *Sociology of Health & Illness*, 28(2), 178–202.

McGlynn, E.A., et al. (2003). The quality of health care delivered to adults in the United States. *New England Journal of Medicine*, 348, 2,635–45.

McIntyre, N. and Popper, K. (1983). The critical attitude in medicine: The need for a new ethics. *British Medical Journal*, 287(24–31 December), 1,919–23.

McKelvie, R.S., et al. (2011). The 2011 Canadian Cardiovascular Society Heart Failure Management Guidelines Update: Focus on sleep apnea, renal dysfunction, mechanical circulatory support, and palliative care. *Canadian Journal of Cardiology*, 27, 319–38.

McLoughlin, V., et al. (2006). Selecting indicators for patient safety at the health system level in OECD countries. *International Journal for Quality in Health Care*, 18(Suppl. 1), 14–20.

McMahon, J., MacCurtain, S. and O'Sullivan, M. (2010). Bullying, culture, and climate in health care organizations: A theoretical framework. In J. Braithwaite, P. Hyde and C. Pope (eds), *Culture and Climate in Health Organizations*. Basingstoke: Palgrave Macmillan (pp. 82–96).

McWhiter, J.J., et al. (2007). *At Risk Youth: A Comprehensive Response for Counselors, Teachers, Psychologists and Human Service Professionals* (4th Edition). Belmont, CA: Thomson.

Meadows, D. (1999). Leverage points: Places to intervene in a system. *Solutions*, 1(1), 41–9.

Meadows, D.H., Meadows, D.L. and Randers, J. (1992). *Beyond the Limits: Global Collapse or a Sustainable Future.* London: Earthscan Publications Ltd.

Meadows, K.A. (2011). Patient-reported outcome measures: An overview. *British Journal of Community Nursing*, 16(3), 146–51.

Melchers, R.E. (2001). On the ALARP approach to risk management. *Reliability Engineering & System Safety*, 71(2), 201–8.

Mennin, S. (2010). Self-organisation, integration and curriculum in the complex world of medical education. *Medical Education*, 44(1), 20–30.

Merton, R.K. (1936). The unanticipated consequences of social action. *American Sociological Review*, 1, 894–904.

Mesman, J. (2009). The geography of patient safety: A topical analysis of sterility. *Social Science & Medicine*, 69(12), 1,705–12.

Mesman, J. (2011). Resources of strength: An exnovation of hidden competencies to preserve patient safety. In E. Rowley, and J. Waring (eds), *A Socio-Cultural Perspective on Patient Safety*. Aldershot, UK: Ashgate.

Michel, P., et al. (2004). Comparison of three methods for estimating rates of adverse events and rates of preventable adverse events in acute care hospitals. *British Medical Journal*, 328, 1–5.

Miller, D. (1993). The architecture of simplicity. *Academy of Management Review*, 18, 116–38.

Milne, J. (2012). Junior doctors' understanding and reenactment of interprofessional learning and practice: A study of international medical graduates in Australian teaching hospitals. Unpublished PhD thesis. University of New South Wales .

Milovanovich, C. (2008). *Inquest into the Death of Vanessa Ann Anderson*. Westmead File No. 161/2007. Sydney: NSW Coroner's Court, Westmead.

Moen, R. and Norman, C. (2012). *Evolution of the PDCA Cycle*. Online at http://www.pkpinc.com/files/NA01MoenNormanFullpaper.pdf, accessed 22 June 2012.

Morel, G., Amalberti, R. and Chauvin, C. (2008). Articulating the differences between safety and resilience: The decision-making of professional sea fishing skippers. *Human Factors*, 1, 1–16.

Nabhan, M., et al. (2012). What is preventable harm in healthcare? A systematic review of definitions. *BMC Health Services Research*. 12, 128.

Narusawa, T. and Shook, J. (2009). *Kaizen Express: Fundamentals for Your Lean Journey*. Cambridge, MA: Lean Enterprise Institute, Inc.

National Health Service. (2012). *National Health Service Institute for Innovation and Improvement Medical Leadership Competency Framework*. Online at http://www.institute.nhs.uk/assessment_tool/general/medical_leadership_competency_framework_-_homepage.html, accessed 31 August 2012.

National Patient Safety Agency. (2008). *Haemodialysis Patients: Risks Associated with Water Supply (Hydrogen Peroxide)*. Online at http://www.nrls.npsa.nhs.uk/resources/?EntryId45=59893, accessed 18 August 2012.

Neuman, H.B., Charlson, M.E. and Temple, L.K. (2007). Is there a role for decision aids in cancer-related decisions? *Critical Review of Oncology / Hematology*, 62, 240–50.

Newhouse, I., et al. (2012). Barriers to the management of heart failure in Ontario long-term care homes: An interprofessional care perspective. *Journal of Research in Interprofessional Education and Practice*, 2(3), 278–95.

Nicolini, D., Waring, J. and Mengis, J. (2011). Policy and practice in the use of root cause analysis to investigate clinical adverse events: Mind the gap. *Social Science & Medicine*, 73(2), 217–25.

Nugus, P. (2008). The interactionist self and grounded research: Reflexivity in a study of emergency department clinicians. *Qualitative Sociology Review*, 4(1), 189–204.

Nugus, P. and Braithwaite, J. (2010). The dynamic interaction of quality and efficiency in the emergency department: Squaring the circle? *Social Science & Medicine*, 70(4), 511–17.

Nugus, P., et al. (2010). Integrated care in the emergency department: A complex adaptive systems perspective. *Social Science & Medicine*, 17(11), 1,997–2,004.

Nyssen, A.S. (2007). Coordination in hospitals: Organized or emergent process? *Cognition, Technology & Work*, 9(3), 149–57.

Nyssen, A.S. and Javaux, D. (1996). Analysis of synchronization constraints and associated errors in collective work environments. *Ergonomics*, 39, 1,249–64.

O'Connor, P., et al. (2012). An evaluation of the effectiveness of the crew resource management programme in naval aviation. *International Journal of Human Factors and Ergonomics*, 1(1), 21–40.

O'Daniel, M. and Rosenstein, A. (2008). Professional communication and team collaboration. In R. Hughes (ed.), *Patient Safety and Quality: An Evidence-Based Handbook for Nurses*. Rockville, MD: Agency for Healthcare Research and Quality.

O'Leary, V.E. and Bhaju, J. (2006). Resilience and empowerment. In J. Worell and C. D. Goodheart (eds), *Handbook of Girls' and Women's Psychological Health: Gender and Well-Being Across the Lifespan*. New York, NY: Oxford University Press (pp. 157–65).

OECD. (2011). Health expenditure in relation to GDP. In *Health at a Glance 2011: OECD Indicators*. OECD Publishing. Online at http://www.oecd-ilibrary.org/social-issues-migration-health/health-at-a-glance-2011_health_glance-2011-en, accessed 30 August 2012.

Ostrom, E. (2010). Beyond markets and states: Polycentric governance of complex economic systems. *American Economic Review*, 100, 641–72.

Øvretveit, J. and Klazinga N. (2008). *Guidance on Developing Quality and Safety Strategies with a Health System Approach*. World Health Organization.

Online at http://www.euro.who.int/__data/assets/pdf_file/0011/96473/E91317.pdf, accessed 30 August 2012.

Paget, M.A. (1988). *The Unity of Mistakes*. Philadelphia, PA: Temple University Press.

Pahl-Wostl, C. (1997). Dynamic structure of a food web model: Comparison with a food chain model. *Ecological Modelling*, 100(1–3), 103–23.

Pariès, J. (2011). Lessons from the Hudson. In E. Hollnagel, et al. (eds), *Resilience Engineering in Practice: A Guidebook*. Farnham, UK: Ashgate.

Pariès, J. (2012). Palestra Internacional: O desafio do inesperado: a engenharia de resiliencia consegue dar a resposta adequada? Paper presented to the Jornada International Abergo, Rio de Janeiro, Brazil, 21–23 August.

Parker, M. (2000). *Organisational Culture and Identity*. London: Sage.

Patterson, E.S. (2008). Structuring flexibility: The potential good, bad and ugly in standardization of handovers. *Quality & Safety in Health Care*, 17, 4–5.

Pereira, D. (2013). Opening the 'black box' of Human Resource Management's association with team characteristics and performance in healthcare: Lessons from rehabilitation services in public hospitals. Unpublished PhD thesis. University of New South Wales.

Perrow, C. (1967). Framework for the comparative analysis of organizations. *American Sociological Review*, 32(2), 194–208.

Perrow, C. (1984). *Normal Accidents: Living With High Risk Technologies*. New York, NY: Basic Books.

Perrow, C. (1986). *Complex Organizations: A Critical Essay* (3rd edition). New York, NY: Random House.

Perrow, C. (1999). *Normal Accidents: Living with High-Risk Technologies*. Princeton, NJ: Princeton University Press.

Persell, S., et al. (2012). Frequency of inappropriate medical exceptions to quality measures. *Annals of Internal Medicine*. 152, 225–31.

Pham, J.C., et al. (2010). ReCASTing the RCA: An improved model for performing root cause analyses. *American Journal of Medical Quality*, 25, 186–91.

Plaisant, C., et al. (2008). Searching electronic health records for temporal patterns in patient histories: A case study with Microsoft Amalga. *AMIA Annual Symposium*, 601.

Plumb, J. (2012). Professional conceptualisation and accomplishment of patient safety in mental health care. Unpublished PhD thesis., University of New South Wales.Sydney, Australia: University of New South Wales.

Plumb, J., et al. (2011). Professional conceptualisation and accomplishment of patient safety in mental health care: An ethnographic approach. *BMC Health Services Research*, 11[online]. Retrieved 29 August 2012 from http://www.biomedcentral.com/content/pdf/1472-6963-11-100.pdf.

Pollitt, C. (1990). Doing business in the temple: Managers and quality assurance in public services. *Public Administration*, 68(4), 435–42.

Power, M. (2007). *Organized Uncertainty. Designing a World of Risk Management*. Oxford: Oxford University Press.

Pratt Hopp, F., Thornton, N. and Martin, L. (2010). The lived experience of heart failure at the end of life: A systematic literature review. *Health & Social Work*, 35(2), 109–117.

Price, J. (2004). Educating the healthcare professional for capability. In D. Kernick (ed.), *Complexity and Healthcare Organization: A View from the Street*. Oxford: Radcliffe Medical Press (pp. 227–40).

Pronovost, P., et al. (2006a). An intervention to decrease catheter-related bloodstream infections in the ICU. *New England Journal of Medicine*, 355(26), 2,725–32.

Pronovost, P.J., et al. (2006b). Creating high reliability in healthcare organizations. *Health Services Research*, 41(4 Pt 2), 1,599–617.

Radnor, Z.J., Holweg, M. and Waring, J. (2012). Lean in healthcare: The unfilled promise? *Social Science & Medicine*, 74(3), 364–71.

Raduma-Tomàs, M.A., et al. (2011). Doctors' handovers in hospitals: A literature review. *BMJ Quality & Safety*, 20, 128–33.

Rasmussen, J. (1997). Risk management in a dynamic society: A modeling problem, *Safety Science*, 27, 183–213.

Rasmussen, J. and Jensen, A. (1974). Mental procedures in real-life tasks: A case study of electronic troubleshooting, *Ergonomics*, 17, 293–307.

Reason, J.T. (1979). Actions not as planned: The price of automatization. In G. Underwood and R. Stevens (eds), *Aspects of Consciousness*. Vol. I, *Psychological Issues*. London: Academic Press.

Reason, J.T. (1990). *Human Error*. Cambridge: Cambridge University Press.

Reason, J.T. (1993). The identification of latent organizational failures in complex systems. In J.A. Wise, D.V. Hopkin and P. Stager (eds), *Verification and Validation of Complex Systems: Human Factors Issues*. Berlin: Springer Verlag.

Reason, J.T. (1997). *Managing the Risks of Organizational Accidents*. Aldershot, UK: Ashgate.

Reason, J.T. (2008). *The Human Contribution*. Farnham, UK: Ashgate.

Repenning, N.P. and Sterman, J.D. (2001). Nobody ever gets credit for fixing problems that never happened: Creating and sustaining process improvement. *California Management Review*, 43(4), 64–88.

Resar, R. (2007). Discussion about the conflation of quality and safety in health care (Personal communication, March, 2007).

Riegel, B., et al. (2009). State of the science: Promoting self-care in persons with heart failure: A scientific statement from the American Heart Association. *Circulation*, 120, 1,141–63.

Rittel, H. and Webber, M. (1973). Dilemmas in a general theory of planning, *Policy Sciences*, 4, 155–169,

Rivard, P.E., Rosen, A.K. and Carroll, J.S. (2006). Enhancing patient safety through organizational learning: Are patient safety indicators a step in the right direction? *Health Service Research*, 41(4), 1,633–53.

Rizzo, J.R., House, R.J. and Lirtzman, S.I. (1970). Role conflict and ambiguity in complex organizations. *Administrative Science Quarterly*, 15(2), 150–63.

Roberts, K.H. (1990). Some characteristics of one type of high reliability organization. *Organization Science*, 1(2), 160–76.

Roberts, K.H., et al. (2005). A case of the birth and death of a high reliability healthcare organisation. *Quality and Safety in Health Care*, 14, 216–20.

Roberts, K.H., Stout, S.K. and Halpern, J.T. (1994). Decision dynamics in two high reliability military organizations. *Management Science*, 40, 614–24.

Rochlin, G.I. (1999). Safe operation as a social construct. *Ergonomics*, 42(11), 1,549–60.

Rochlin, G.I., La Porte, T.R. and Roberts, K.H. (1987). Self-designing high reliability: Aircraft carrier flight operations at sea. *Naval War College Review*, 40(4), 76–90.

Rosenthal, M. (1995). *The Incompetent Doctor*. Buckingham: Open University Press.

Roshanov, P.S., et al. (2011). Computerized clinical decision support systems for chronic disease management: A decision-maker-researcher partnership systematic review. *Implementation Science*, 6, 92.

Rowley, E. and Waring, J. (eds.), (2011). *A Socio-Cultural Perspective on Patient Safety*. Farnham, UK: Ashgate.

Rudolph, J.W., Morrison, J.B. and Carroll, J.S. (2009). The dynamics of action-oriented problem solving: Linking interpretation and choice. *Academy of Management Review*, 34(4), 733–56.

Runciman, W.B., et al. (2012a). CareTrack: Assessing the appropriateness of health care delivery in Australia. *Medical Journal of Australia*, 197(2), 100–105.

Runciman, W.B., et al. (2012b). Towards the delivery of appropriate health care in Australia. *Medical Journal of Australia*, 197(2), 78.

Ryder, M., et al. (2011). Multidisciplinary heart failure management and end of life care. *Current Opinion in Supportive and Palliative Care*, 4, 317–21.

Salas, E., et al. (2008). Does team training work? Principles for health care. *Academic Emergency Medicine*, 15(11), 1,002–9.

Salas, E., et al. (2006). Does crew resource management training work? An update, an extension, and some critical needs. *Human Factors*, 48(2), 392–412.

Sanne J.M. (2008). Incident reporting or storytellling? Competing schemes in a safety-critical and hazardous work setting. *Safety Science*, 46, 1,205–22.

Savoyant, A. and Leplat J. (1983), Statut et fonction des communications dans l'activité des équipes de travail. *Psychologie Française*, 28(3), 247–53.

Scarpello, J. (2010). After the abolition of the National Patient Safety Agency. *British Medical Journal*, 341, 1,005–6.

Schein, E. (2004). *Organizational Culture and Leadership*. San Francisco: Jossey-Bass.

Schmidt, D.C., Corsaro, A. and van't Hag, H. (2008). Addressing the challenges of tactical information management in net-centric systems with DDS. *CrossTalk: The Journal of Defense Software Engineering* (March), 24–9.

Schulman, P.R. (1993). Analysis of high reliability organizations: A comparative framework. In K.H. Roberts (ed.), *New Challenges to Understanding Organizations*. New York, NY: Macmillan.

Schulman, P.R. (2004). General attributes of safe organizations. *Quality and Safety in Health Care*, 13(Suppl. II), ii39–ii44.

Schuur, J.D. and Venkatesh, A.K. (2012). The growing role of emergency departments in hospital admissions. *New England Journal of Medicine*, 367(5), 391–3.

Senge, P.M. (2006). *The Fifth Discipline: The Art and Practice of the Learning Organization*. Revised and updated. New York: Doubleday / Currency.

Shaw, C.D., Jelfs, E. and Franklin, P. (2012). Implementing recommendations for safer hospitals in Europe: Sanitas Project. *Eurohealth*, 18(2), 26–8.

Simon, H.A. (1947). *Administrative Behavior: A Study of Decision-Making Processes in Administrative Organization* (1st Edition). New York: Macmillan.

Simon, H.A. (1955). A behavioral model of rational choice. *Quarterly Journal of Economics*, 69, 99–118.

Simon, H.A. (1956). Rational choice and the structure of the environment. *Psychological Review*, 63(2), 129–38.

Simon, H.A. (1979). Rational decision-making in business organizations. *American Economic Review*, 69, 493–513.

Sjohania, K.., et al. (2007). How quickly do systematic reviews go out of date? A survival analysis. *Annals of International Medicine*, 147, 224–33.

Skinner, C.A., et al. (2009). Reforming New South Wales public hospitals: An assessment of the Garling inquiry. *Medical Journal of Australia*, 190(2), 78–9.

Smetzer, J. and Cohen, M. (1998). Lessons from the Denver medication error / criminal negligence case: Look beyond blaming individuals. *Hospital Pharmacy*, 33, 640–56.

Smircich, L. (1983). Concepts of culture and organizational analysis. *Administrative Science Quarterly*, 28(3), 339–58.

Smit, B. and Wandel, J. (2006). Adaptation, adaptive capacity and vulnerability. *Global Environmental Change: Human and Policy Dimensions*, 16(3), 282–92.

Snook, S.A. (2000). *Friendly Fire*. Princeton and Oxford: Princeton University Press.

Solow, L. and Fake, B. (2010). *What Works for GE May Not Work for You*. New York, NY: Productivity Press.

Stacey, R.D. (1992). *Managing the Unknowable: Strategic Boundaries between Order and Chaos in Organizations*. San Francisco: Jossey-Bass.

Stewart, G.J. and Dwyer, J.M. (2010). Implementation of the Garling recommendations can offer real hope for rescuing the New South Wales public hospital system. *Medical Journal of Australia*, 190(2), 80.

Storey, N. (1996). *Safety-Critical Computer Systems*. Harlow: Pearson Education Limited.

Strachan, P.H., et al. (2009). Mind the Gap: Opportunities for improving end-of-life care for patients with advanced heart failure. *The Canadian Journal of Cardiology*, 25(11), 635–40.

Strauss, A.L. (1978). *Negotiations: Varieties, Contexts, Processes, and Social Order*. San Francisco: Jossey-Bass.

Strauss, A.L., et al. (1963). The hospital and its negotiated order. In E. Freidson (ed), *The Hospital in Modern Society*. London: Free Press of Glencoe (pp. 147–69).

Sutcliffe, K.M., Lewton, E. and Rosenthal, M.M. (2004). Communication failures: An insidious contributor to medical mishaps. *Academic Medicine*, 79(2), 186–94.

Sutcliffe, K.M. and Vogus, T.J. (2003). Organizing for resilience. In K.S. Cameron, and J.E. Dutton (eds), *Positive Organizational Scholarship: Foundations of a New Discipline*. London: Berrett-Koehler.

Syer, C.A., et al. (2003). Adaptive-creative versus routine-reproductive expertise in hypermedia design: An exploratory study. *Cognition, Technology & Work*, 5, 94–106.

Szalay, A. and Gray, J. (2006). 2020 computing: Science in an exponential world. *Nature*, 440(7,083), 413 14.

Szulanski, G. (2003). *Sticky Knowledge: Barriers to Knowing in the Firm*. London: Sage.

Tague, N.R. (2004). *The Quality Toolbox* (2nd Edition). Milwaukee: ASQ Quality Press, 390–92.

Tassaux, D., et al. (2008). Evolution des soins intensifs en Suisse: historique, situation actuelle et perspectives. *Revue Médicale Suisse*, 4(183), pp. 2,672–6.

The New York Times (2010). *Factory Efficiency Comes to the Hospital* (10 July). Online at http://www.nytimes.com/2010/07/11/business/11seattle.html?pagewanted=all&_r=0, accessed 25 October 2012.

Thomas, E., Sexton, J. and Helmreich, R. (2004). Translating teamwork behaviours from aviation to healthcare: Development of behavioural markers for neonatal resuscitation. *Quality and Safety in Health Care*, 13, 57–64.

Thompson, R.F. and Spencer, W.A. (1966). Habituation: A model phenomenon for the study of neuronal substrates of behavior. *Psychological Review*, 73(1), 16–43.

Timmermans, S. and Berg, M. (2003). *The Gold Standard: The Challenge of Evidence-Based Medicine and Standardization in Health Care*. Philadelphia, PA: Temple University Press.

Travaglia, J.F., Westbrook, M.T. and Braithwaite, J. (2009). Implementation of a patient safety incident management system as viewed by doctors, nurses and allied health professionals. *Health*, 13(3), 277–96.

Tucker, A.L. (2010). *The Workaround Culture: Unintended Consequences of Organizational Heroes*. Havard Business School Working Knowledge. Retrieved 8 November 2012, from http://hbswk.hbs.edu/item/6572.html?wknews=110810.

Tucker, A.L. and Edmondson, A.C. (2002). When problem solving prevents organizational learning. *Journal of Organizational Change Management*, 15(2), 122 –37.

Tucker, A.L. and Edmondson, A.C. (2003). Why hospitals don't learn from failures: Organizational and psychological dynamics that inhibit system change. *California Management Review*, 45(2), 55–72.

Ungar, M. (2006). *Strengths-based Counseling for At-risk Youth*. Thousand Oaks, CA: Corwin Press.

Ungar, M. (2008). Resilience across cultures. *British Journal of Social Work*, 38(2), 218–35.

Valderas, J.M., Alonso, J. and Guyatt, G.H. (2008). Measuring patient-reported outcomes: Moving from clinical trials into clinical practice. *Medical Journal of Australia*, 189, 93–4.

Verschaffel, L., Torbeyns, J. and Van Dooren, W. (2009). Conceptualizing, investigating, and enhancing adaptive expertise in mathematics education. *European Journal of Psychology of Education*, XXIV(3), 335–59.

Vincent, C. (1993). The study of errors and accidents in medicine. In C. Vincent, M. Ennis and R. Audley (eds), *Medical Accidents*. Oxford: Oxford University Press.

Vincent, C. (2010). *Patient Safety* (2nd Edition). Oxford: Wiley Blackwell.

Vincent, C., et al. (2008). Is health care getting safer? *British Medical Journal*, 337(7,680), 1,205–7.

Vincent, C., Benn, J. and Hanna, G.B. (2010). High reliability in health care. *British Medical Journal*, 340, c84.

Vogus, T.J. (2004). In search of mechanisms: How do HR practices affect organizational performance? Doctoral dissertation. University of Michigan.

Vogus, T.J. and Sutcliffe, K.M. (2007a). The safety organizing scale: Development and validation of a behavioral measure of safety culture in hospital nursing units. *Medical Care*, 45(1), 46–54.

Vogus, T.J. and Sutcliffe, K.M. (2007b). The impact of safety organizing, trusted leadership, and care pathways on reported medication errors in hospital nursing units. *Medical Care*, 45(10), 997–1,002.

Wachter, R. (2010). Patient safety at ten: Unmistakable progress, troubling gaps. *Health Affairs*, 29(1), 165–73.

Waldrop, M.M. (1992). *Complexity: The Emerging Science at the Edge of Order and Chaos*. New York: Simon and Shuster.

Walker, B., et al. (2004). Resilience, adaptability and transformability in social-ecological systems. *Ecology and Society*, 9(2), 5.

Walshe, K. (2003). *Regulating Healthcare: A Prescription for Improvement?* Maidenhead: Open University Press.

Waring, J. (2005). Beyond blame: The cultural barriers to medical incident reporting. *Social Science & Medicine*, 60, 1,927–35.

Waring, J. (2007a). Getting to the roots of patient safety. *International Journal of Quality in Healthcare*, 19(5), 257–8.

Waring, J. (2007b). Adaptive regulation or governmentality: Patient safety and the changing regulation of medicine. *Sociology of Health and Illness*, 29(2), 163–79.

Waring, J. (2010). Critical risk management: Moral entrepreneurship in the pursuit of patient safety. In G. Currie, et al. (eds), *Critical Public Sector Management*. London: Routledge.

Waring, J., Harrison, S. and McDonald, R. (2007). A culture of safety or coping: Ritualistic behaviours in the operating department. *Journal of Health Services Research and Policy*, 12(1, Suppl. 1), 3–9.

Waring, J., McDonald, R. and Harrison, S. (2006). Safety and complexity: The inter-departmental threats to patient safety in the operating department. *Journal of Health, Organisation and Management*, 20(3), 227–42.

Waring, J., et al. (2010). A narrative review of the UK Patient Safety Research Portfolio. *Journal of Health Services Research and Policy*, 15(1, Suppl. 2), 26–32.

Wears, R.L. and Cook, R.I. (2010). Getting better at doing worse. *Annals of Emergency Medicine*, 56(5), 465–67.

Wears, R.L. and Perry, S.J. (2006). 'Free fall' – A case study of resilience, its degradation, and recovery, in an emergency department. Paper presented at the 2nd International Symposium on Resilience Engineering, Juan-les-Pins, France. Online at http://www.resilience-engineering.org/REPapers/Wears_et_al.pdf.

Wears, R.L. and Webb, L.K. (2011). Fundamental or situational surprise: A case study with implications for resilience. Presented at the 4th Resilience Engineering Symposium. Sophia Antipolis, France, 8–10 June.

Weick, K.E. (1979). *The Social Psychology of Organizing* (2nd Edition). New York: McGraw-Hill.

Weick, K.E. (1987). Organizational culture as a source of high reliability. *California Management Review*, 29(2), 112–27.

Weick, K.E. (1995). *Sense-Making in Organizations*. London: Sage.

Weick, K.E. (1998). Enacted sense-making in crisis situations. *Journal of Management Studies*, 25(4), 305–17.

Weick, K.E. (2011). Organizing for transient reliability: The production of dynamic non-events. *Journal of Contingencies and Crisis Management*, 19(1), 21–7.

Weick, K.E. and Roberts, K.H. (1993). Collective mind in organizations: Heedful interrelating on flight decks. *Administrative Science Quarterly*, 38(3), 357–81.

Weick, K.E. and Sutcliffe, K.M. (2006). Mindfulness and the quality of organizational attention. *Organization Science*, 17(4), 514–24.

Weick, K.E. and Sutcliffe, K.M. (2007). *Managing the Unexpected: Resilience Performance in an Age of Uncertainty* (2nd Edition). San Francisco, CA: Jossey-Bass.

Weick, K.E., Sutcliffe, K.M. and Obstfeld, D. (1999). Organizing for high reliability: Processes of collective mindfulness. In B.M. Staw and L.I. Cummings (eds), *Research in Organizational Behavior*. Greenwich, CT: JAI Press (pp. 81–123).

Wellman, J., Jeffries, H. and Hagan, P. (2011). *Leading the Lean Healthcare Journey: Driving Culture Change to Increase Value*. New York, NY: Productivity Press.

Westrum, R. (1994). Thinking by groups, organizations and networks: A sociologist's view of the social psychology of science and technology. In W.R. Shadish and S. Fuller (eds), *The Social Psychology of Science*. NY: Guilford Press (pp. 329–39).

Westrum, R. (2006). A typology of resilience situations. In E. Hollnagel, D.D. Woods and N. Leveson (eds), *Resilience Engineering: Concepts and Precepts*. Aldershot, UK: Ashgate. (pp. 55–65.)

WHO Collaborating Centre for Patient Safety Solutions (2007). *Communication During Patient Hand-Overs, Patient Safety Solutions*, 1, 1–4. Online at http://www.ccforpatientsafety.org/common/pdfs/fpdf/presskit/PS-Solution3.pdf, accessed 28 July 2012.

Wiegmann, D.A. and Shappell, S.A. (1999). Human error and crew resource management failures in naval aviation mishaps: A review of US Naval Safety Center data, 1990–96. *Aviation, Space, and Environmental Medicine*, 70(12), 1,147–51.

Wildavsky, A. (1988). *Searching for Safety*. Berkeley, CA: University of California Press.

Wilson, R.M., et al. (1999). An analysis of the causes of adverse events from the Quality in Australian Health Care Study. *Medical Journal of Australia*, 170(9), 411–15.

Windle, G., Bennett, K. and Noyes, J. (2011). A methodological review of resilience measurement scales. *BMC Health and Quality of Life Outcomes*, 9(8).

Woloschynowych, M., et al. (2005). The investigation and analysis of critical incidents and adverse events in healthcare. *Health Technologies Assessment*, 9(19).

Woods, D.D. (2003). *Creating Foresight: How Resilience Engineering Can Transform NASA's Approach to Risk Decision-Making*. US Senate Testimony for the Committee on Commerce, Science and Transportation, John McCain, chair. Washington, D.C., 29 October 2003.

Woods, D.D. (2006). Essential characteristics of resilience. In E. Hollnagel, D.D. Woods and N. Leveson (eds), *Resilience Engineering: Concepts and Precepts*. Aldershot, UK: Ashgate (pp. 21–33).

Woods, D.D. (2010). Resilience and the ability to anticipate. In E. Hollnagel, et al. (eds), *Resilience Engineering in Practice: A Guidebook*. Farnham, UK: Ashgate.

Woods, D.D. and Branlat, M. (2011a). Basic patterns in how adaptive systems fail. In E. Hollnagel, et al. (eds), *Resilience Engineering in Practice: A Guidebook*. Farnham, UK: Ashgate.

Woods, D.D. and Branlat, M. (2011b). How human adaptive systems balance fundamental trade-offs: Implications for polycentric governance architectures. Presented at the 4th International Conference on Resilience Engineering. Sophia Antipolis, France.

Woods, D.D. and Hollnagel, E. (2006). *Joint Cognitive Systems: Patterns in Cognitive Systems Engineering*. Boca Raton, FL: CRC Press / Taylor and Francis Group.

Woods, D.D. and Shattuck, L.G. (2000). Distant supervision – Local action given the potential for surprise. *Cognition, Technology & Work*, I, 86–96.

World Alliance for Patient Safety (2005). WHO draft guidelines for adverse event reporting and learning systems. Online at http://www.who.int/patientsafety/events/05/Reporting_Guidelines.pdf, accessed 22 June 2012.

Wu, W., Lipshutz, K.M. and Pronovost, P.J. (2008). Effectiveness and efficiency of root cause analysis in medicine. *Journal of the American Medical Association*, 299, 685–7.

Zhao, L., et al. (2011). Herd behavior in a complex adaptive system. *Proceedings of the National Academy of Science USA*, 108(37), 15,058–63.

Zimmerman, B. Lindberg, C. and Plsek, P. (1998). *Edgeware: Lessons from Complexity Science for Health Care Leaders*. Santa Fe, NM: Plexus Institute.

Index